THE COMPLETE GALVESTON DIET COOKBOOK FOR BEGINNERS

1200 Days of Wholesome and Mouthwatering Recipes to Live a Healthier Lifestyle, Featuring

Seasonal Ingredients and Creative Twists on Classic Dishes| Full-Color Picture Premium Edition

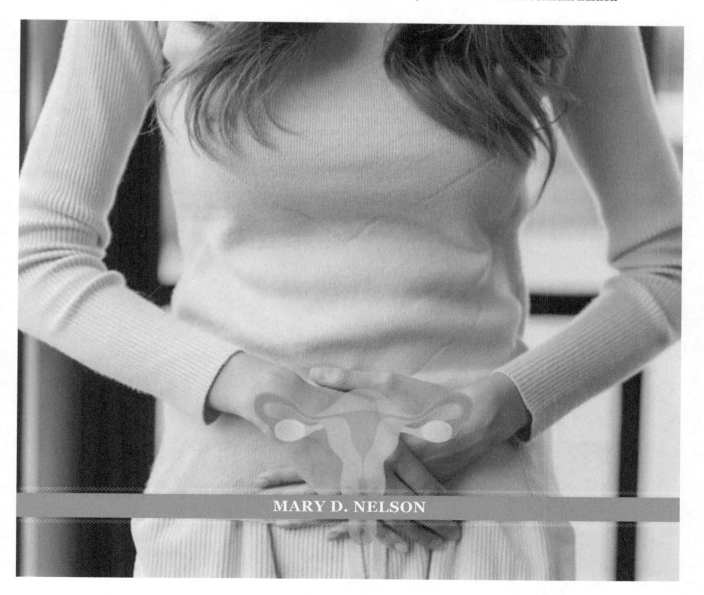

MARY D. NELSON

EDITOR: LYN   INTERIOR DESIGN: FAIZAN

COVER ART: ABR   FOOD STYLIST: JO

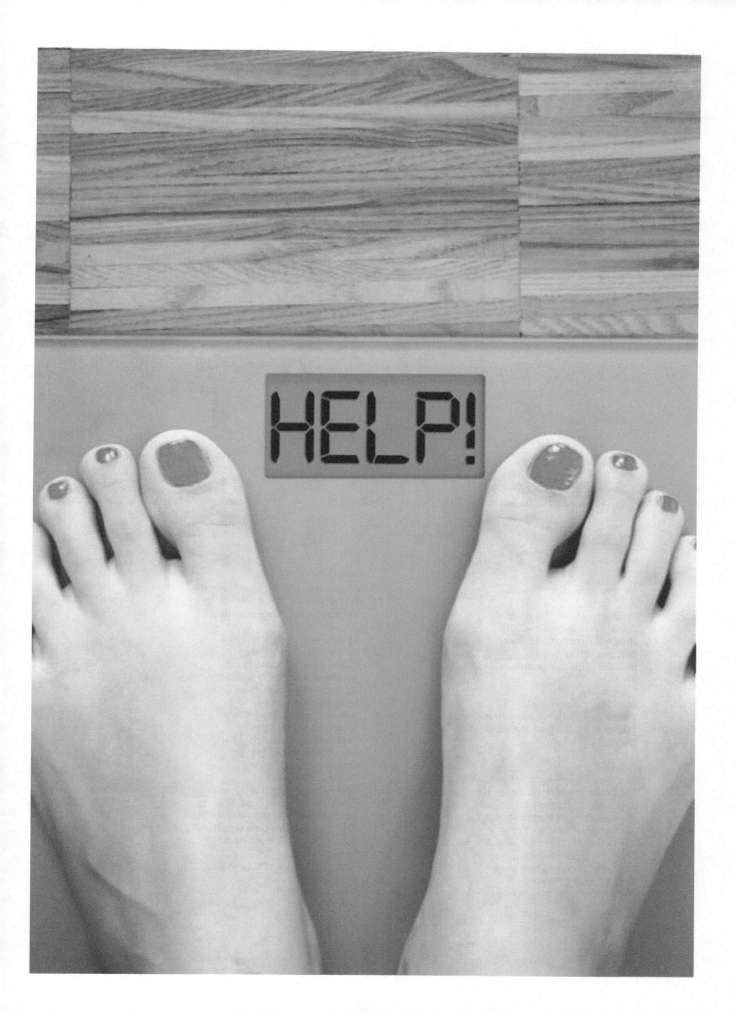

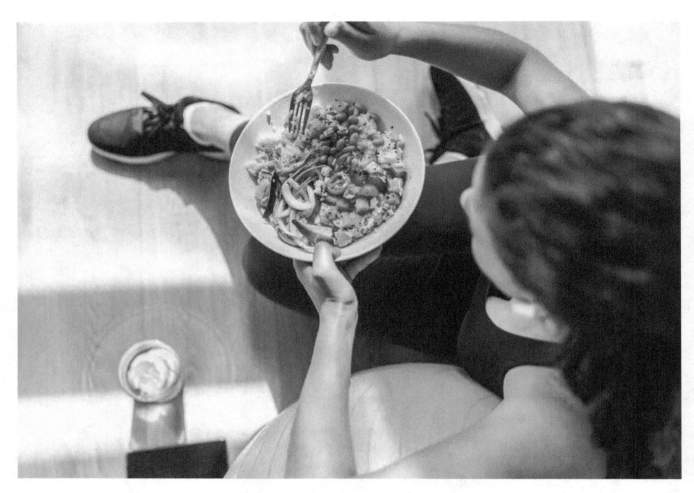

Table of Contents

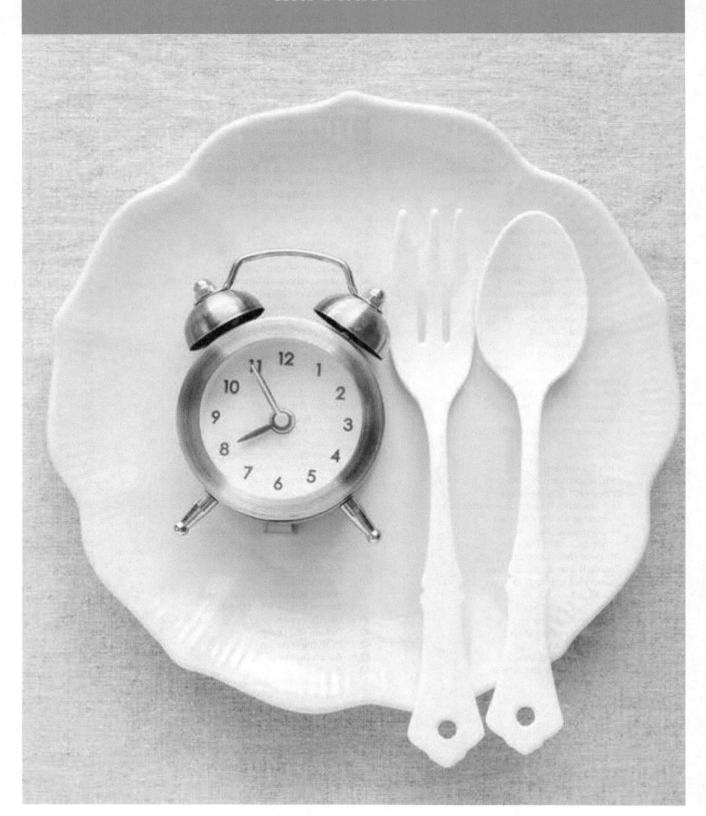

Women go through a variety of changes in midlife that can be challenging to navigate. Hormonal fluctuations, changes in metabolism, and lifestyle factors can all contribute to weight gain, inflammation, and other health issues. However, there are steps that women can take to support their health and wellbeing during this time.

The Galveston diet is a program designed specifically for women over 40 who are experiencing the changes of midlife. It emphasizes the importance of balanced nutrition, regular exercise, and self-care to support hormonal balance, reduce inflammation, and promote weight loss.

Polycystic ovary syndrome (PCOS) is a common endocrine disorder that affects many women of childbearing age. It's estimated that around 1 in 10 women have PCOS, and the majority of them are overweight or obese.

PCOS is characterized by a variety of symptoms, including irregular periods, elevated levels of androgens (male hormones), and the formation of multiple cysts on the ovaries. These symptoms can make it difficult for women with PCOS to conceive, and they may also contribute to weight gain and other health issues.

Maintaining a healthy weight is important for women with PCOS, as excess weight can exacerbate symptoms and increase the risk of complications such as diabetes, high blood pressure, and heart disease. The Galveston diet program may be helpful for women with PCOS who are looking to lose weight and improve their overall health. By following a balanced, nutrient-dense diet and incorporating regular exercise and self-care, women with PCOS can support their health and wellbeing and manage the symptoms of their condition.

By following the Galveston diet program and incorporating healthy habits into their daily routine, women can feel more confident and in control of their health as they navigate the changes of midlife. Whether you're looking to shed a few pounds, reduce inflammation, or simply feel better overall, the Galveston diet can provide the guidance and support you need to reach your health goals.

Chapter 1
The Galveston Diet and You

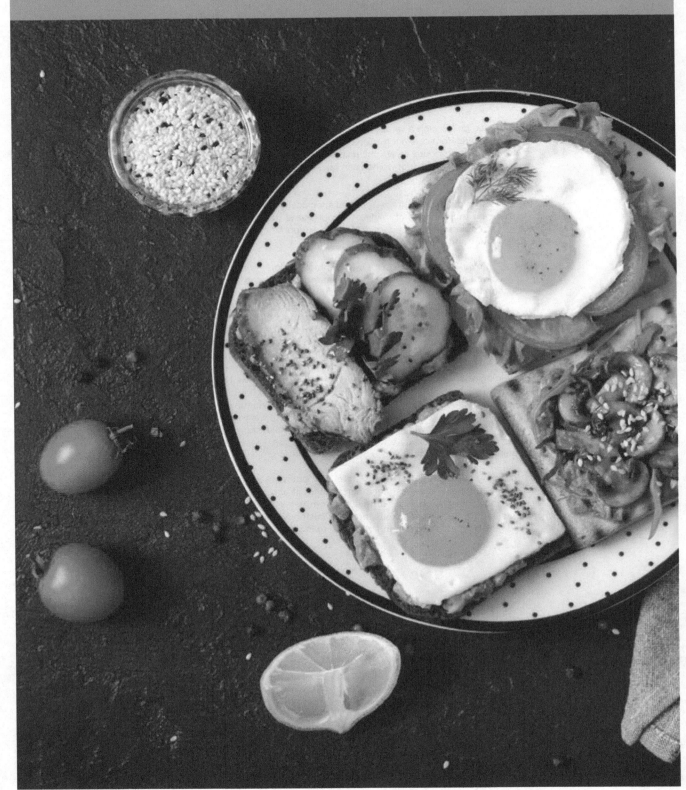

What is Galveston Diet?

The Galveston diet is a weight loss program designed specifically for women over the age of 40. It was created by Dr. Mary Claire Haver, an OB-GYN in Galveston, Texas. The program focuses on balancing hormones through nutrition and exercise to help women lose weight, reduce inflammation, and improve overall health.

The Galveston diet involves a combination of intermittent fasting and a low-carbohydrate, high-fat (LCHF) diet. The fasting aspect of the diet involves limiting food intake to a specific time frame each day, usually between 12-16 hours. During the eating window, the focus is on consuming healthy, nutrient-dense foods such as whole grains, fruits, vegetables, lean proteins, and healthy fats.

The Galveston diet also emphasizes the importance of exercise, particularly resistance training, for maintaining muscle mass and increasing metabolism. The program also encourages women to prioritize self-care and stress reduction through activities such as yoga, meditation, and adequate sleep.

It's important to note that while the Galveston diet may be effective for some women, it's always a good idea to consult with a healthcare professional before starting any new diet or exercise program.

Changes in Your Body

PERIMENOPAUSE

Postmenopause is a stage of life that begins after a woman has gone 12 consecutive months without a menstrual period. During this time, the body undergoes a variety of changes, including a decrease in estrogen levels and changes in metabolism that can contribute to weight gain and other health issues.

Research suggests that cells may store more fat and be slower to release it during postmenopause, which can make weight management more challenging. However, adopting healthy lifestyle habits such as regular exercise, balanced nutrition, and stress management can help women in postmenopause maintain a healthy weight and support their overall health and wellbeing.

The Galveston diet program may be particularly beneficial for women in postmenopause, as it is designed to support hormonal balance, reduce inflammation, and promote weight loss. By following the program's recommendations for balanced nutrition, regular exercise, and self-care, women in postmenopause can support their health and feel their best as they navigate this new stage of life. It's important to consult with a healthcare professional before starting any new diet or exercise program, particularly if you have a medical condition or are taking medications.

MENOPAUSE

Menopause is the stage of life during which a woman's ovaries stop producing reproductive hormones, resulting in the cessation of menstrual periods. It is typically diagnosed after a woman has gone 12 consecutive months without a period.

The average age of menopause is 51, but it is normal for women to experience it as early as their mid-40s or as late as their mid-50s. The onset of menopause can be influenced by a variety of factors, including genetics, lifestyle, and underlying medical conditions.

During menopause, women may experience a range of symptoms such as hot flashes, mood changes, and vaginal dryness, which can impact their quality of life. However, adopting healthy lifestyle habits such as regular exercise, balanced nutrition, and stress management can help women manage their symptoms and support their overall health and wellbeing.

POSTMENOPAUSE

Postmenopause is a stage of life that begins after a woman has gone 12 consecutive months without a menstrual period. During this time, the body undergoes a variety of changes, including a decrease in estrogen levels and changes in metabolism that can contribute to weight gain and other health issues.

Research suggests that cells may store more fat and be slower to release it during postmenopause, which can make weight management more challenging. Postmenopausal women are also at higher risk of developing visceral fat, which is a type of fat that accumulates around the internal organs and can increase the risk of chronic diseases such as type 2 diabetes, heart disease, and certain cancers.

Adopting healthy lifestyle habits such as regular exercise, balanced nutrition, and stress management can help women in postmenopause maintain a healthy weight and support their overall health and wellbeing. The Galveston diet program may be particularly beneficial for postmenopausal women, as it is designed to support hormonal balance, reduce inflammation, and promote weight loss.

By following the program's recommendations for balanced nutrition, regular exercise, and self-care, women in postmenopause can support their health and reduce their risk of chronic diseases.

Benefits of the Galveston Diet

The Galveston Diet can offer a range of benefits for women, especially those who are in perimenopause, menopause, or postmenopause. Here are some of the benefits:

1. Weight loss: The Galveston Diet can help women lose weight, particularly in the abdominal area, where it is most important to reduce visceral fat. It does this by encouraging the body to utilize fat for fuel, and by limiting foods that promote inflammation and weight gain.
2. Reduced inflammation: By cutting out inflammatory foods and consuming anti-inflammatory foods, the Galveston Diet can help to reduce inflammation in the body. This, in turn, can alleviate symptoms of chronic disease, including joint pain and stiffness.
3. Improved energy: With the Galveston Diet, you'll be consuming healthy fats that can provide sustained energy throughout the day. This can help to reduce fatigue and boost mental clarity.
4. Reduced menopausal symptoms: By eliminating inflammatory foods and focusing on whole, nutrient-dense foods, the Galveston Diet can help to reduce hot flashes, night sweats, and other symptoms of menopause.
5. Reduced risk of chronic disease: The Galveston Diet promotes a healthy eating pattern that includes plenty of fruits, vegetables, lean protein, and healthy fats. This eating pattern has been shown to reduce the risk of chronic diseases, such as heart disease, diabetes, and cancer.
6. Improved gut health: The Galveston Diet encourages the consumption of fiber-rich foods, which can help to promote healthy digestion and improve gut health.

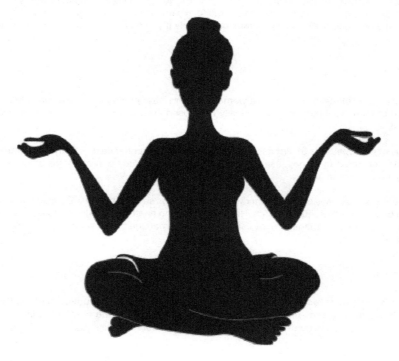

Chapter 2
Start to Change Your Life

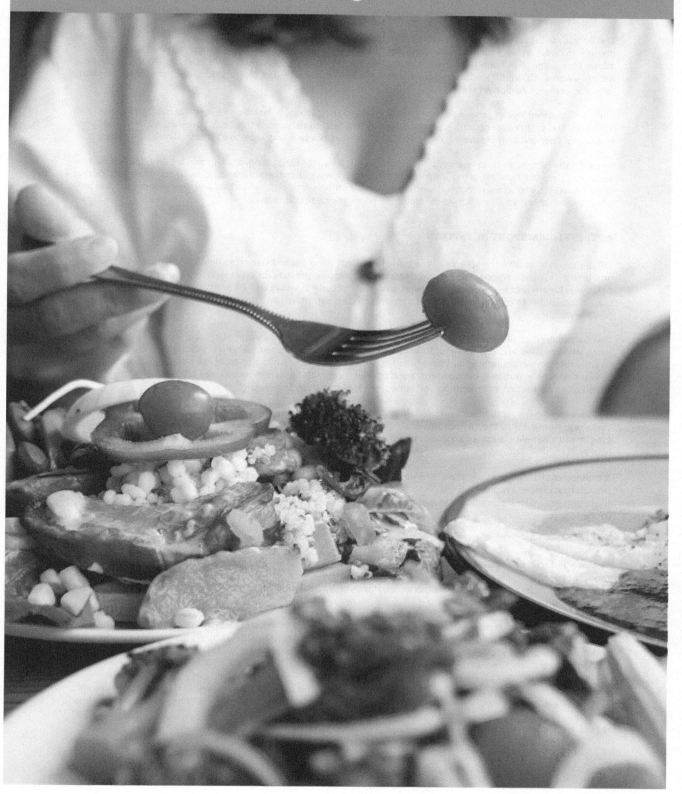

Three Key Actions Involved in the Galveston Diet

INTERMITTENT FASTING

Intermittent Fasting is a key component of the Galveston Diet, especially for women in menopause. Intermittent Fasting involves periods of time where you do not eat, typically ranging from 12 to 16 hours. During this period, the body shifts from using glucose as its primary source of energy to burning stored fat. The result is improved insulin sensitivity and increased fat burning, which can contribute to weight loss and improved overall health.

The Galveston Diet program recommends a 16:8 Intermittent Fasting approach, which involves fasting for approximately 16 hours a day, including overnight, and then eating within a consecutive 8-hour window. This approach allows for a balance between fasting and eating, making it easier to maintain for most people. During the 8-hour eating window, it's important to consume balanced, nutrient-dense meals that include adequate protein, healthy fats, and complex carbohydrates.

While Intermittent Fasting may seem intimidating at first, many people find it to be an easy habit to develop and maintain. The program encourages gradually extending fasting periods as the body becomes more accustomed to the practice, and also provides guidance on how to break the fast and what to eat during the eating window.

Overall, Intermittent Fasting is a key component of the Galveston Diet program and can be an effective tool for supporting weight loss, reducing inflammation, and promoting hormonal balance in women, especially during menopause. It's important to consult with a healthcare professional before starting any new diet or exercise program, particularly if you have a medical condition or are taking medications.

ANTI-INFLAMMATORY NUTRITION

Inflammation is a natural response of the body to protect itself against harmful stimuli, such as infection, injury, and toxins. However, when inflammation becomes chronic and persists for an extended period of time, it can lead to various health problems, including weight gain and difficulty in losing weight. Women in menopause are particularly susceptible to inflammation, which can worsen their symptoms and make it more challenging to maintain a healthy weight.

The Galveston Diet program emphasizes anti-inflammatory nutrition by eliminating or reducing foods that promote inflammation and encouraging foods that fight it. Highly processed carbohydrates, added sugars, and unhealthy fats are particularly inflammatory and should be avoided or limited as much as possible. Instead, the diet focuses on whole, nutrient-dense foods, such as fruits, vegetables, whole grains, lean proteins, and healthy fats, which can help reduce inflammation and support overall health and wellbeing.

By following the Galveston Diet's anti-inflammatory nutrition principles, women in menopause can reduce the severity and frequency of their symptoms and achieve a healthy weight. Not only that, but they may also experience other health benefits, such as improved blood sugar control, reduced risk of chronic diseases, and improved gut health.

It's important to note that adopting an anti-inflammatory diet should be part of a comprehensive lifestyle approach that includes regular exercise, stress management, and adequate sleep. By addressing multiple factors that contribute to inflammation and menopausal symptoms, women can improve their overall health and quality of life.

FUEL REFOCUS

The Fuel Refocus phase of the Galveston Diet is all about adjusting the ratio of macronutrients in your diet to promote fat burning and prevent fat storage. When you consume a carbohydrate-heavy diet, your body burns those calories for energy and stores any excess as fat. However, by depleting your carb intake, your body is forced to turn to other sources for fuel, such as fat.

During the Fuel Refocus phase, you'll be encouraged to consume a diet rich in healthy fats, lean protein, and complex carbohydrates. By following the recommended ratio of 70 percent healthy fats, 20 percent lean protein, and 10 percent carbohydrates, you can shift your body's metabolism to rely more on fat for fuel, leading to improved weight loss and overall health.

Healthy fats, such as those found in nuts, seeds, avocados, and fatty fish, are essential for maintaining healthy hormone levels and promoting satiety. Lean protein sources, such as chicken, fish, and legumes, can help build and repair muscle tissue and promote a feeling of fullness. Complex carbohydrates, such as those found in whole grains and vegetables, provide essential nutrients and fiber to support overall health.

By adjusting your macronutrient ratio and focusing on healthy fats, lean protein, and complex carbohydrates, you can optimize your body's ability to burn fat and improve your health and wellbeing. The Fuel Refocus phase is an essential part of the Galveston Diet program and can help women in menopause achieve their weight loss goals and improve their overall health.

Tips for Following the Galveston Diet

Tips can be very important for successfully following the Galveston Diet or any other diet plan. Tips can provide guidance, motivation, and inspiration for making lifestyle changes and sticking to a healthy eating plan. They can also help you avoid common mistakes and pitfalls and make the transition to a new way of eating easier and more enjoyable.

HERE ARE SOME TIPS FOR FOLLOWING THE GALVESTON DIET:

1. Start with a plan: Take some time to research and plan out your meals for the week. This will help you stay on track and avoid making unhealthy choices.
2. Prepare your meals in advance: Meal prepping is a great way to ensure you have healthy meals ready to eat throughout the week. You can cook large batches of food and portion them out for the week.
3. Focus on whole, unprocessed foods: Eating a diet that is rich in whole, unprocessed foods is one of the best ways to improve your health. These foods are nutrient-dense and can help keep you feeling full and satisfied.
4. Keep healthy snacks on hand: Snacking on unhealthy foods can quickly derail your diet. Keep healthy snacks like fruits, nuts, and vegetables on hand for when you get hungry between meals.
5. Stay hydrated: Drinking plenty of water is essential for good health. Aim for at least 8-10 glasses of water per day.
6. Get enough sleep: Getting enough sleep is important for overall health and can also help with weight loss. Aim for at least 7-8 hours of sleep per night.
7. Stay active: Regular exercise is key to maintaining a healthy weight and improving overall health. Find an activity you enjoy and aim for at least 30 minutes of exercise per day.
8. Monitor your progress: Keep track of your progress by taking measurements and tracking your weight loss. This can help you stay motivated and on track with your goals.
9. Seek support: Join a support group or find a friend who is also following the Galveston Diet. Having someone to share your journey with can make a big difference in your success.

Q&As

HOW DOES INTERMITTENT FASTING WORK?
Intermittent fasting involves fasting for approximately 16 hours a day and then eating within an 8-hour window. This helps to optimize fat burning and decrease insulin resistance.

WHAT TYPES OF FOODS ARE ALLOWED ON THE GALVESTON DIET?
The Galveston Diet emphasizes whole, nutrient-dense foods that are low in added sugars and processed carbo-hydrates, and high in healthy fats, fiber, and protein. Here are some examples of foods that are allowed on the Galveston Diet:

- Healthy fats: avocado, olive oil, coconut oil, nuts, seeds, fatty fish
- Lean proteins: chicken, turkey, fish, seafood, eggs, grass-fed beef and other meats
- Non-starchy vegetables: leafy greens, broccoli, cauliflower, Brussels sprouts, asparagus, peppers, onions, mushrooms, zucchini, squash
- Low-sugar fruits: berries, citrus fruits, apples, pears, kiwi, melons
- Whole grains and legumes (in moderation): quinoa, brown rice, lentils, chickpeas, black beans, kidney beans

- Herbs, spices, and seasonings: garlic, ginger, turmeric, cinnamon, cumin, oregano, rosemary, thyme

CAN I STILL DRINK COFFEE WHILE ON THE GALVESTON DIET?

Yes, you can still drink coffee while on the Galveston Diet. However, it is recommended that you limit your intake of coffee and other caffeinated beverages, as caffeine can increase inflammation and disrupt your sleep. Additionally, it is best to avoid adding sugar or artificial sweeteners to your coffee, and instead use natural sweeteners like stevia or monk fruit extract.

IS EXERCISE NECESSARY WHILE ON THE GALVESTON DIET?

While exercise is not mandatory on the Galveston Diet, it is recommended as it can have numerous health benefits such as improving cardiovascular health, increasing muscle mass, and boosting metabolism. Incorporating regular exercise into your routine can also enhance weight loss efforts and help you maintain a healthy weight. However, it is important to note that the Galveston Diet focuses primarily on nutrition and does not require a specific exercise regimen.

CAN MEN FOLLOW THE GALVESTON DIET?

Yes, men can follow the Galveston Diet. While the diet was originally designed for women in perimenopause and menopause, the principles of the diet can be applied to anyone looking to improve their health and nutrition. The diet emphasizes anti-inflammatory whole foods, healthy fats, and intermittent fasting, which can benefit both men and women. The recommended macronutrient ratio of 70% healthy fats, 20% lean protein, and 10% complex carbohydrates can also be adjusted to suit individual needs and preferences.

CAN I STILL EAT OUT WHILE ON THE GALVESTON DIET?

Yes, you can still eat out while on the Galveston Diet. However, it is important to make smart choices when selecting your meal. Look for options that are rich in healthy fats, lean protein, and non-starchy vegetables. Avoid foods that are high in added sugars, refined carbohydrates, and unhealthy fats.

HERE ARE SOME TIPS FOR EATING OUT ON THE GALVESTON DIET:

- Choose a salad with a variety of colorful vegetables and a protein source such as grilled chicken, fish, or tofu. Opt for oil and vinegar dressing instead of creamy dressings.
- Select a grilled or broiled fish or meat dish and substitute starchy sides like rice or potatoes with non-starchy vegetables.
- Ask for sauces and dressings on the side so you can control how much you consume.
- Avoid fried foods, breaded meats, and creamy sauces, which tend to be high in unhealthy fats and calories.
- Drink water or unsweetened tea instead of sugary drinks like soda or sweetened iced tea.

Remember, the Galveston Diet is all about making sustainable lifestyle changes, so don't feel like you have to deprive yourself of social events and dining out. Just make sure to make healthy choices whenever possible.

HOW LONG DOES IT TAKE TO SEE RESULTS ON THE GALVESTON DIET?

Results on the Galveston Diet may vary depending on factors such as your starting weight, age, metabolism, and adherence to the diet. Some people may see noticeable changes in their weight and symptoms within the first few weeks of following the diet, while for others it may take longer. It's important to remember that the Galveston Diet is not a quick fix, but a sustainable lifestyle change. By following the diet consistently and making it a part of your daily routine, you can achieve long-term benefits for your health and well-being.

In conclusion, the Galveston Diet is a comprehensive plan designed specifically for women who are going through perimenopause, menopause, and postmenopause. It emphasizes intermittent fasting, anti-inflammatory nutrition, and fuel refocusing to help women achieve and maintain a healthy weight and improve their overall health and well-being.

By following the guidelines and tips provided in the Galveston Diet, women can expect to see significant improvements in their weight, energy levels, mood, and overall health within a matter of weeks. However, it is important to note that the Galveston Diet is not a quick-fix solution, but rather a lifestyle change that requires commitment and dedication.

With caution and proper guidance, the Galveston Diet can be a beneficial and effective approach to managing menopausal symptoms and improving overall health for women.

Chapter 3
The Meal Plans and Shopping Lists

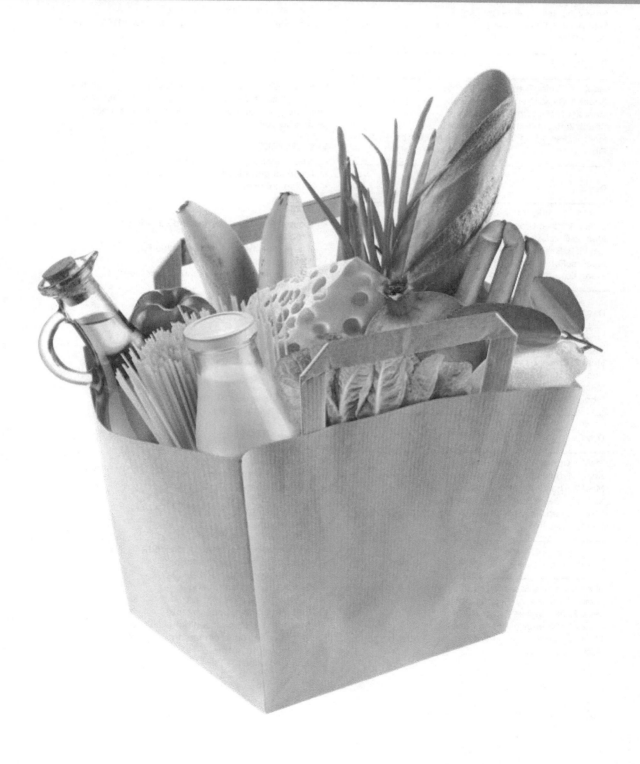

Day 1

Meal 1: Morning Berry-Green Smoothie
Snack 1: Basic Orange Cheesecake
Meal 2: Chicken Creamy Soup
Snack 2: Basic Orange Cheesecake
Macros: Fat: 93.6g, Protein: 35.9g, Net Carbs: 15.3g, Fiber: 0.4g

Day 2

Meal 1: Morning Berry-Green Smoothie
Snack 1: Basic Orange Cheesecake
Meal 2: Chicken Creamy Soup
Snack 2: Basic Orange Cheesecake
Macros: Fat: 93.6g, Protein: 35.9g, Net Carbs: 15.3g, Fiber: 0.4g

Day 3

Meal 1: Morning Berry-Green Smoothie
Snack 1: Basic Orange Cheesecake
Meal 2: Chicken Creamy Soup
Snack 2: Basic Orange Cheesecake
Macros: Fat: 93.6g, Protein: 35.9g, Net Carbs: 15.3g, Fiber: 0.4g

Day 4

Meal 1: Morning Berry-Green Smoothie
Snack 1: Basic Orange Cheesecake
Meal 2: Chicken Creamy Soup
Snack 2: Basic Orange Cheesecake
Macros: Fat: 93.6g, Protein: 35.9g, Net Carbs: 15.3g, Fiber: 0.4g

Day 5

Meal 1: Creamy Sesame Bread
Snack 1: Basic Orange Cheesecake
Meal 2: Thai Sweet Potato Soup
Snack 2: Basic Orange Cheesecake
Macros: Fat: 103.5g, Protein: 24.6g, Net Carbs: 98.2g, Fiber: 11.3g

Day 6

Meal 1: Creamy Sesame Bread
Snack 1: Blueberry-Peach Cobbler
Meal 2: Thai Sweet Potato Soup
Snack 2: Blueberry-Peach Cobbler
Macros: Fat: 91.3g, Protein: 29g, Net Carbs: 113g, Fiber: 30g

Day 7

Meal 1: Creamy Sesame Bread
Snack 1: Blueberry-Peach Cobbler
Meal 2: Thai Sweet Potato Soup
Snack 2: Blueberry-Peach Cobbler
Macros: Fat: 91.3g, Protein: 29g, Net Carbs: 113g, Fiber: 30g

Shopping List for Week 1

Note: Amounts given here indicate the quantities you need for the week's recipes; they are not always indicative of the quantities in which the items are commonly sold.

VEGETABLES
- 3 large sweet potatoes, cubed
- Fresh ginger, sliced (1/2-inch piece)
- 4 tbsp chopped cilantro

FRUITS
- 3 cups mixed blueberries and strawberries
- 2 tablespoons orange juice
- 3 large peaches, peeled and sliced
- 1 avocado, pitted and sliced
- 1/2 cup unsweetened coconut, shredded
- Zest of 1 lime
- Juice of 1 lime

PROTEINS
- 2 cups cooked and shredded chicken
- 4 eggs
- 4 cups chicken broth

NUTS
- 1 cup nuts and seeds mix
- 1 tbsp sesame seeds

MISCELLANEOUS
- 2 cups unsweetened almond milk
- ½ cup cream cheese
- 17 ounces mascarpone cream
- 3 tablespoons Swerve
- 1 cup almond flour
- 1 cup coconut flour
- 2 tsp erythritol
- 2 tbsp psyllium husk powder
- 5 tablespoons coconut oil, divided
- 1 teaspoon powdered gelatin
- 1 tablespoon maple syrup
- 1 tablespoon coconut sugar
- ½ teaspoon vanilla extract
- Salt and black pepper, to taste
- 1 teaspoon salt, plus additional as needed
- 1 teaspoon ground cinnamon
- Pinch ground nutmeg
- 1 cup ice cubes

Day 1

Meal 1: Breakfast Naan Bread
Snack 1: Coconut Cranberry Bars
Meal 2: Cream of Thyme Tomato Soup
Snack 2: Coconut Cranberry Bars
Macros: Fat: 72.2g, Protein: 19.4g, Net Carbs: 14.6g,
Fiber:8.8g

Day 2

Meal 1: Breakfast Naan Bread
Snack 1: Coconut Cranberry Bars
Meal 2: Cream of Thyme Tomato Soup
Snack 2: Coconut Cranberry Bars
Macros: Fat: 72.2g, Protein: 19.4g, Net Carbs: 14.6g,
Fiber:8.8g

Day 3

Meal 1: Breakfast Naan Bread
Snack 1: Coconut Cranberry Bars
Meal 2: Cream of Thyme Tomato Soup
Snack 2: Coconut Cranberry Bars
Macros: Fat: 72.2g, Protein: 19.4g, Net Carbs: 14.6g,
Fiber:8.8g

Day 4

Meal 1: Breakfast Naan Bread
Snack 1: Coconut Cranberry Bars
Meal 2: Cream of Thyme Tomato Soup
Snack 2: Coconut Cranberry Bars
Macros: Fat: 72.2g, Protein: 19.4g, Net Carbs: 14.6g,
Fiber:8.8g

Day 5

Meal 1: Breakfast Naan Bread
Snack 1: Coconut Cranberry Bars
Meal 2: Cream of Thyme Tomato Soup
Snack 2: Coconut Cranberry Bars
Macros: Fat: 72.2g, Protein: 19.4g, Net Carbs: 14.6g,
Fiber:8.8g

Day 6

Meal 1: Breakfast Naan Bread
Snack 1: Coconut Cranberry Bars
Meal 2: Cream of Thyme Tomato Soup
Snack 2: Coconut Cranberry Bars
Macros: Fat: 72.2g, Protein: 19.4g, Net Carbs: 14.6g,
Fiber:8.8g

Day 7

Meal 1: Tuna Caprese Salad
Snack 1: Iced Vanilla Coconut Latte
Meal 2: Tuna Caprese Salad
Snack 2: Iced Vanilla Coconut Latte
Macros: Fat: 132.6g, Protein:48.8g, Net Carbs:14.6g,
Fiber:10.6g

Shopping List for Week 2

VEGETABLES
- 2 garlic cloves
- 2 large red onions
- 4 tomatoes
- 6 basil leaves

FRUITS
- 1/3 cup cranberries
- 1/2 lemon

PROTEINS
- 2 cans (10 oz each) Tuna chunks in water, drained

NUTS
- 1/2 cup raw cashew nuts

MISCELLANEOUS
- 3/4 cup almond flour
- 2 tbsp psyllium husk powder
- 1/2 tsp baking powder
- 3 tbsp olive oil
- 4 oz peanut butter
- 2 tbsp ghee
- 1/2 cup butter, melted
- 1/2 teaspoon liquid stevia
- 1/2 cup black olives, pitted and sliced
- 1 cup coconut milk, unsweetened
- 4 tablespoons coconut cream
- 1/2 cup brewed black coffee
- a pinch of grated nutmeg
- a pinch of ground cinnamon
- 1 vanilla bean

The Conventional Menus: Week 3

Day 1

Meal 1: Pork and Cheddar Sausages
Snack 1: Peanut and Butter Cubes
Meal 2: Salmon & Asparagus Skewers
Snack 2: Peanut and Butter Cubes
Macros: Fat: 77.4g, Protein: 64.6g, Net Carbs: 14.2g, Fiber: 12.4g

Day 2

Meal 1: Pork and Cheddar Sausages
Snack 1: Peanut and Butter Cubes
Meal 2: Salmon & Asparagus Skewers
Snack 2: Peanut and Butter Cubes
Macros: Fat: 77.4g, Protein: 64.6g, Net Carbs: 14.2g, Fiber: 12.4g

Day 3

Meal 1: Pork and Cheddar Sausages
Snack 1: Peanut and Butter Cubes
Meal 2: Salmon & Asparagus Skewers
Snack 2: Peanut and Butter Cubes
Macros: Fat: 77.4g, Protein: 64.6g, Net Carbs: 14.2g, Fiber: 12.4g

Day 4

Meal 1: Pork and Cheddar Sausages
Snack 1: Peanut and Butter Cubes
Meal 2: Salmon & Asparagus Skewers
Snack 2: Peanut and Butter Cubes
Macros: Fat: 77.4g, Protein: 64.6g, Net Carbs: 14.2g, Fiber: 12.4g

Day 5

Meal 1: Pork and Cheddar Sausages
Snack 1: Peanut and Butter Cubes
Meal 2: Salmon & Asparagus Skewers
Snack 2: Peanut and Butter Cubes
Macros: Fat: 77.4g, Protein: 64.6g, Net Carbs: 14.2g, Fiber: 12.4g

Day 6

Meal 1: Pork and Cheddar Sausages
Snack 1: Mediterranean Tahini Beans
Meal 2: Salmon & Asparagus Skewers
Snack 2: Mediterranean Tahini Beans
Macros: Fat: 45g, Protein: 60g, Net Carbs: 34g, Fiber: 13g

Day 7

Meal 1: Pork and Cheddar Sausages
Snack 1: Mediterranean Tahini Beans
Meal 2: Salmon & Asparagus Skewers
Snack 2: Mediterranean Tahini Beans
Macros: Fat: 45g, Protein: 60g, Net Carbs: 34g, Fiber: 13g

Shopping List for Week 3

VEGETABLES:
- 1 pound asparagus spears
- 1 cup string beans, trimmed

FRUITS:
- 2 lemons

PROTEINS:
- 2½ pounds pork butt
- 1½ pounds boned skinless salmon
- ½ cup peanuts, toasted and coarsely chopped

MISCELLANEOUS:
- 1 stick butter (8 tablespoons)
- 1/3 cup coconut oil
- ½ pound pork fat
- 2 tablespoons Monk fruit powder
- 1 tablespoon lard or coconut oil
- 2 tablespoons ghee, melted
- 2 feet medium hog casings
- 2 cups finely diced sharp cheddar cheese
- 2 tablespoons pure tahini
- 2 tablespoons chopped mint leaves
- 1/4 teaspoon cinnamon powder
- 1 teaspoon Dijon mustard
- 1 teaspoon garlic powder
- ¼ teaspoon red chili flakes
- Sea salt to taste
- 1 tablespoon fine sea salt
- 1 vanilla paste
- ¼ cup chopped green onions or 2 tablespoons dried chives

Day 1

Meal 1: Lamb Meatballs with Dill Sauce
Snack 1: Easiest Brownies Ever
Meal 2: Chicken Bone Broth
Snack 2: Peanut Butter and Chocolate Treat
Macros: Fat: 49.2g, Protein: 25.2g, Net Carbs: 12.3g,
Fiber: 5.2g

Day 2

Meal 1: Lamb Meatballs with Dill Sauce
Snack 1: Easiest Brownies Ever
Meal 2: Chicken Bone Broth
Snack 2: Peanut Butter and Chocolate Treat
Macros: Fat: 49.2g, Protein: 25.2g, Net Carbs: 12.3g,
Fiber: 5.2g

Day 3

Meal 1: Lamb Meatballs with Dill Sauce
Snack 1: Easiest Brownies Ever
Meal 2: Chicken Bone Broth
Snack 2: Peanut Butter and Chocolate Treat
Macros: Fat: 49.2g, Protein: 25.2g, Net Carbs: 12.3g,
Fiber: 5.2g

Day 4

Meal 1: Lamb Meatballs with Dill Sauce
Snack 1: Easiest Brownies Ever
Meal 2: Chicken Bone Broth
Snack 2: Peanut Butter and Chocolate Treat
Macros: Fat: 49.2g, Protein: 25.2g, Net Carbs: 12.3g,
Fiber: 5.2g

Day 5

Meal 1: Lamb Meatballs with Dill Sauce
Snack 1: Easiest Brownies Ever
Meal 2: Chicken Bone Broth
Snack 2: Peanut Butter and Chocolate Treat
Macros: Fat: 49.2g, Protein: 25.2g, Net Carbs: 12.3g,
Fiber: 5.2g

Day 6

Meal 1: Lamb Meatballs with Dill Sauce
Snack 1: Easiest Brownies Ever
Meal 2: Chicken Bone Broth
Snack 2: Peanut Butter and Chocolate Treat
Macros: Fat: 49.2g, Protein: 25.2g, Net Carbs: 12.3g,
Fiber: 5.2g

Day 7

Meal 1: Lamb Meatballs with Dill Sauce
Snack 1: Easiest Brownies Ever
Meal 2: Chicken Bone Broth
Snack 2: Peanut Butter and Chocolate Treat
Macros: Fat: 49.2g, Protein: 25.2g, Net Carbs: 12.3g,
Fiber: 5.2g

Shopping List for Week 4

VEGETABLES:

- 2 carrots
- 1 celery stalk
- ½ onion

PROTEINS:

- 1½ pounds ground lamb
- 1 chicken carcass
- 4 eggs
- 1/4 cup pork rinds

MISCELLANEOUS:

- 1 cup Avocado-Dill Sauce
- 2 tablespoons almond flour
- 3 tablespoons coconut flour
- 1/2 cup cocoa powder, unsweetened
- 1/2 cup Swerve
- 1 teaspoon almond extract
- 1 vanilla extract
- 1/2 cup coconut oil
- 3 ounces baking chocolate, unsweetened
- 1 stick butter, room temperature
- 1/3 cup peanut butter
- 1/3 cup unsweetened coconut flakes
- Bay leaves
- Parsley sprig
- Garlic cloves
- Dried oregano
- Dried basil leaves
- Ground cumin
- Pumpkin pie spice
- Paprika
- Freshly ground black pepper
- Sea salt
- Apple cider vinegar

The Vegetarian Menus: Week 1

Day 1

Meal 1: Pumpkin Muffins
Snack 1: Traditional Spanish Frisuelos
Meal 2: Chickpea and Kale Salad
Snack 2: Seedy Cookie Dough Bites
Macros: Fat: 50.3g, Protein: 37.1g, Net Carbs: 99.2g, Fiber: 17g

Day 2

Meal 1: Pumpkin Muffins
Snack 1: Traditional Spanish Frisuelos
Meal 2: Chickpea and Kale Salad
Snack 2: Seedy Cookie Dough Bites
Macros: Fat: 50.3g, Protein: 37.1g, Net Carbs: 99.2g, Fiber: 17g

Day 3

Meal 1: Pumpkin Muffins
Snack 1: Traditional Spanish Frisuelos
Meal 2: Chickpea and Kale Salad
Snack 2: Seedy Cookie Dough Bites
Macros: Fat: 50.3g, Protein: 37.1g, Net Carbs: 99.2g, Fiber: 17g

Day 4

Meal 1: Pumpkin Muffins
Snack 1: Traditional Spanish Frisuelos
Meal 2: Chickpea and Kale Salad
Snack 2: Seedy Cookie Dough Bites
Macros: Fat: 50.3g, Protein: 37.1g, Net Carbs: 99.2g, Fiber: 17g

Day 5

Meal 1: Pumpkin Muffins
Snack 1: Traditional Spanish Frisuelos
Meal 2: Masala Lentils
Snack 2: Seedy Cookie Dough Bites
Macros: Fat:41.3, Protein:36.1, Net Carbs:96.2, Fiber:20g

Day 6

Meal 1: Pumpkin Muffins
Snack 1: Traditional Spanish Frisuelos
Meal 2: Masala Lentils
Snack 2: Seedy Cookie Dough Bites
Macros: Fat:41.3, Protein:36.1, Net Carbs:96.2, Fiber:20g

Day 7

Meal 1: Masala Lentils
Snack 1: Iced Vanilla Coconut Latte
Meal 2: Masala Lentils
Snack 2: Iced Vanilla Coconut Latte
Macros: Fat: 46.3g, Protein: 15.4g, Net Carbs: 38.3g, Fiber: 16.3g

Shopping List for Vegetarian Week 1

VEGETABLES:
- Kale

FRUITS:
- Lemon
- Pumpkin puree

PROTEINS:
- Chickpeas
- Eggs

NUTS:
- Almond flour
- Cacao nibs
- Gluten-free rolled oats
- Pumpkin seeds
- Sunflower seeds

MISCELLANEOUS:
- Avocado
- Black coffee
- Butter (unsalted)
- Coconut cream
- Coconut milk (unsweetened)
- Cream cheese (8 oz. package)
- Diced tomatoes (15 oz. can)
- Extra-virgin olive oil
- Garam masala
- Garlic powder
- Ground cinnamon
- Ground cloves
- Ground ginger
- Ground nutmeg
- Liquid or powdered sweetener (Swerve confectioners'-style sweetener or equivalent amount)
- Maple syrup
- Molasses
- Paprika (sweet)
- Salt (fine sea salt)
- Vanilla extract
- Vanilla bean
- Vegetable broth
- Cayenne pepper
- Full-fat coconut milk
- Kite Hill brand cream cheese style spread (if dairy-free)

Day 1

Meal 1: Tiramisu Muffins
Snack 1: Classic Chocolate Sheet Cake
Meal 2: Classic Vegetable Broth
Snack 2: Almond Butter and Chocolate Cookies
Macros: Fat: 83.3g, Protein: 28.3g, Net Carbs: 63.4g,
Fiber: 7.7g

Day 2

Meal 1: Tiramisu Muffins
Snack 1: Classic Chocolate Sheet Cake
Meal 2: Classic Vegetable Broth
Snack 2: Almond Butter and Chocolate Cookies
Macros: Fat: 83.3g, Protein: 28.3g, Net Carbs: 63.4g,
Fiber: 7.7g

Day 3

Meal 1: Tiramisu Muffins
Snack 1: Classic Chocolate Sheet Cake
Meal 2: Classic Vegetable Broth
Snack 2: Almond Butter and Chocolate Cookies
Macros: Fat: 83.3g, Protein: 28.3g, Net Carbs: 63.4g,
Fiber: 7.7g

Day 4

Meal 1: Tiramisu Muffins
Snack 1: Classic Chocolate Sheet Cake
Meal 2: Classic Vegetable Broth
Snack 2: Almond Butter and Chocolate Cookies
Macros: Fat: 83.3g, Protein: 28.3g, Net Carbs: 63.4g,
Fiber: 7.7g

Day 5

Meal 1: Tiramisu Muffins
Snack 1: Classic Chocolate Sheet Cake
Meal 2: Classic Vegetable Broth
Snack 2: Almond Butter and Chocolate Cookies
Macros: Fat: 83.3g, Protein: 28.3g, Net Carbs: 63.4g,
Fiber: 7.7g

Day 6

Meal 1: Tiramisu Muffins
Snack 1: Classic Chocolate Sheet Cake
Meal 2: Classic Vegetable Broth
Snack 2: Almond Butter and Chocolate Cookies
Macros: Fat: 83.3g, Protein: 28.3g, Net Carbs: 63.4g,
Fiber: 7.7g

Day 7

Meal 1: Tiramisu Muffins
Snack 1: Classic Chocolate Sheet Cake
Meal 2: Classic Vegetable Broth
Snack 2: Almond Butter and Chocolate Cookies
Macros: Fat: 83.3g, Protein: 28.3g, Net Carbs: 63.4g,
Fiber: 7.7g

Shopping List for Vegetarian Week 2

VEGETABLES:
- 2 garlic cloves
- 1 parsley sprig
- 6 cups veggie scraps (peels and pieces of carrots, celery, onions, garlic)
- ½ medium onion
- 2 bay leaves

PROTEINS:
- 6 large eggs
- 1 (8-ounce) package mascarpone cheese (or Kite Hill brand cream cheese style spread if dairy-free)

FRUITS
- 1 avocado

MISCELLANEOUS:
- ½ cup coconut flour
- 2 cups blanched almond flour
- ½ cup Swerve confectioners'-style sweetener or equivalent amount of liquid or powdered sweetener
- 2 tablespoons unsweetened cocoa powder
- ¼ teaspoon fine sea salt
- ¼ teaspoon baking soda
- ½ cup (1 stick) unsalted butter (or coconut oil if dairy-free)
- ½ cup brewed decaf espresso or other strong brewed decaf coffee
- 2 teaspoons rum extract
- Unsweetened cocoa powder, for dusting
- Olive oil
- 12 cups filtered water
- ¾ teaspoon sea salt
- ½ teaspoon dried oregano
- ½ teaspoon dried basil leaves
- 1/2 teaspoon baking powder
- 1/4 teaspoon ground cinnamon
- 1/4 cup cocoa powder, unsweetened
- 1/3 cup coconut oil
- 1/4 cup powdered erythritol
- 1/2 teaspoon butterscotch extract
- 1/2 cup Monk fruit powder
- 3 cups pork rinds, crushed
- 1 teaspoon vanilla extract
- 1/4 teaspoon ground cinnamon
- 1/2 cup sugar-free chocolate, cut into chunks
- 1/2 cup double cream

Chapter 4
Smoothies & Breakfasts

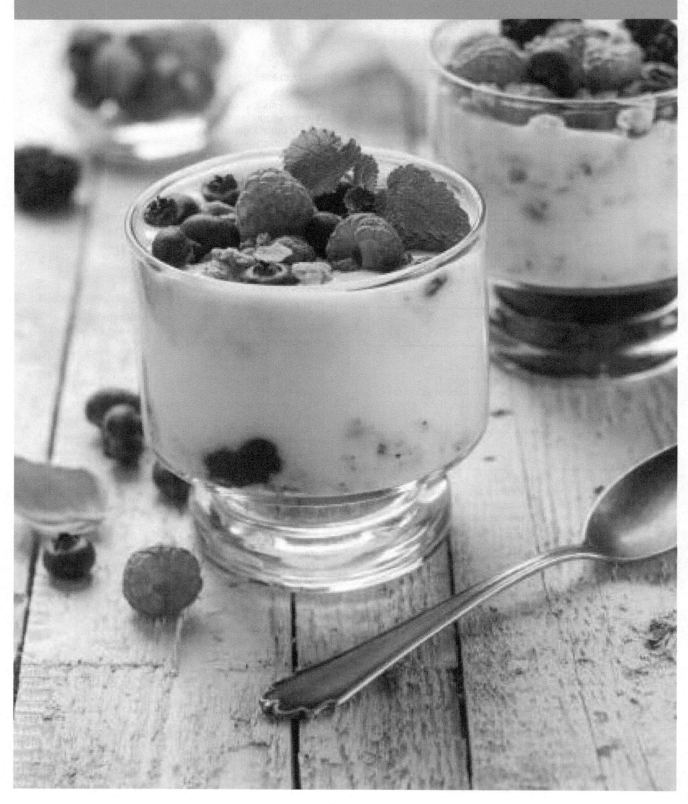

Morning Berry-Green Smoothie

Prep time: 5 minutes | **Cook time:** 5 minutes | **Serves 4**

- 1 avocado, pitted and sliced
- 3 cups mixed blueberries and strawberries
- 2 cups unsweetened almond milk
- 6 tbsp heavy cream
- 2 tsp erythritol
- 1 cup ice cubes
- ⅓ cup nuts and seeds mix

1. Combine the avocado slices, blueberries, strawberries, almond milk, heavy cream, erythritol, ice cubes, nuts and seeds in a smoothie maker; blend in high-speed until smooth and uniform.
2. Pour the smoothie into drinking glasses, and serve immediately.

PER SERVING

Kcal: 360 | Fat: 33.3g | Net Carbs: 6g | Protein: 6g

Breakfast Nut Granola & Smoothie Bowl

Prep time: 5 minutes | **Cook time:** 5 minutes | **Serves 4**

- 6 cups Greek yogurt
- 4 tbsp almond butter
- A handful toasted walnuts
- 3 tbsp unsweetened cocoa powder
- 4 tsp swerve brown sugar
- 2 cups nut granola for topping

1. Combine the Greek yogurt, almond butter, walnuts, cocoa powder, and swerve brown sugar in a smoothie maker; puree in high-speed until smooth and well mixed.
2. Share the smoothie into four breakfast bowls, top with a half cup of granola each, and serve.

PER SERVING

Kcal: 361 | Fat: 31.2g | Net Carbs: 2g | Protein: 13g

Bacon and Egg Quesadillas

Prep time: 30 minutes | **Cook time:** 6 minutes | **Serves 4**

- 8 low carb tortilla shells
- 6 eggs
- 1 cup water
- 3 tbsp butter
- 1 ½ cups grated cheddar cheese
- 1 ½ cups grated Swiss cheese
- 5 bacon slices
- 1 medium onion, thinly sliced
- 1 tbsp chopped parsley

1. Bring the eggs to a boil in water over medium heat for 10 minutes. Transfer the eggs to an ice water bath, peel the shells, and chop them; set aside.
2. Meanwhile, as the eggs cook, fry the bacon in a skillet over medium heat for 4 minutes until crispy. Remove and chop. Plate and set aside too.
3. Fetch out 2/3 of the bacon fat and sauté the onions in the remaining grease over medium heat for 2 minutes; set aside. Melt 1 tablespoon of butter in a skillet over medium heat.
4. Lay one tortilla in a skillet; sprinkle with some Swiss cheese. Add some chopped eggs and bacon over the cheese, top with onion, and sprinkle with some cheddar cheese. Cover with another tortilla shell. Cook for 45 seconds, then carefully flip the quesadilla, and cook the other side too for 45 seconds. Remove to a plate and repeat the cooking process using the remaining tortilla shells.
5. Garnish with parsley and serve warm.

PER SERVING

Kcal: 449 | Fat: 48.7g | Net Carbs: 6.8g | Protein: 29.1g

Breakfast Naan Bread
Prep time: 5 minutes | Cook time: 20 minutes | Serves 6

- ¾ cup almond flour
- 2 tbsp psyllium husk powder
- ½ tsp sea salt
- ½ tsp baking powder
- 3 tbsp olive oil
- 4 oz peanut butter
- 2 garlic cloves, minced

1. In a bowl, mix the almond flour, psyllium husk powder, salt, and baking powder.
2. Mix in some olive oil and 2 cups of boiling water to combine the ingredients, like a thick porridge.
3. Stir and allow the dough to rise for 5 minutes.
4. Divide the dough into 6 to 8 pieces and mold into balls.
5. Place the balls on parchment paper and flatten them with your hands.
6. Warm the peanut butter in a frying pan and fry the naan on both sides to have a beautiful, golden color.
7. Transfer the naan to a plate and keep warm in the oven.
8. For the garlic butter, add the remaining peanut butter to the frying pan and sauté the garlic until fragrant, about 3 minutes.
9. Pour the garlic butter into a bowl and serve as a dip along with the naan.

PER SERVING
Cal 255| Fat 23g| Carbs 6.7g| Protein 7.5g

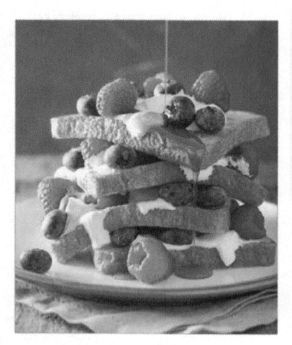

Sweet Potato Pie Smoothie
Prep time: 5 minutes | Cook time: 15 minutes | Serves 2

- ½ cup unsweetened almond milk
- ½ cup freshly squeezed orange juice
- 1 cup cooked sweet potato
- 1 banana
- 2 tablespoons pumpkin seeds
- 1 tablespoon pure maple syrup
- ½ teaspoon pure vanilla extract
- ½ teaspoon ground cinnamon
- 3 ice cubes

1. In a blender, combine the almond milk, orange juice, sweet potato, banana, pumpkin seeds, maple syrup, vanilla, and cinnamon. Blend until smooth.
2. Add the ice and blend until thick.

PER SERVING
Calories: 235 | Total fat: 4g | Saturated Fat: 1g | Carbohydrates: 43g | Fiber: 6g | Protein: 5g

Avocado and Kale Eggs
Prep time: 20 minutes | Cook time: 11 minutes | Serves 4

- 1 tsp ghee
- 1 red onion, sliced
- 4 oz chorizo, sliced into thin rounds
- 1 cup chopped kale
- 1 ripe avocado, pitted, peeled, chopped
- 4 eggs
- Salt and black pepper to season

1. Preheat oven to 370°F.
2. Melt ghee in a cast iron pan over medium heat and sauté the onion for 2 minutes. Add the chorizo and cook for 2 minutes more, flipping once.
3. Introduce the kale in batches with a splash of water to wilt, season lightly with salt, stir and cook for 3 minutes. Mix in the avocado and turn the heat off.
4. Create four holes in the mixture, crack the eggs into each hole, sprinkle with salt and black pepper, and slide the pan into the preheated oven to bake for 6 minutes until the egg whites are set or firm and yolks still runny. Season to taste with salt and pepper, and serve right away with low carb toasts.

PER SERVING
Kcal: 274 | Fat: 23g | Net Carbs: 4g | Protein: 13g

Fruit And Seed Breakfast Bars

Prep time: 15 minutes | Cook time: 30 minutes | Serves 6

- ½ cup pitted dates
- ¾ cup toasted sunflower seeds
- ¾ cup toasted pumpkin seeds
- ¾ cup white sesame seeds
- ½ cup dried blueberries
- ½ cup dried cherries
- ¼ cup flaxseed
- ½ cup almond butter

1. Preheat the oven to 325°F.
2. Line an 8-by-8-inch baking dish with parchment paper.
3. In a food processor, pulse the dates until chopped into a paste.
4. Add the sunflower seeds, pumpkin seeds, sesame seeds, blueberries, cherries, and flaxseed, and pulse to combine. Scoop the mixture into a medium bowl.
5. Stir in the almond butter. Transfer the mixture to the prepared dish and press it down firmly.
6. Bake for about 30 minutes, or until firm and golden brown.
7. Cool for about 1 hour, until it is at room temperature. Remove from the baking dish and cut into 12 squares.
8. Refrigerate in a sealed container for up to 1 week.

PER SERVING

Calories: 312 | Total fat: 22g | Saturated Fat: 4g | Carbohydrates: 24g | Fiber: 6g | Protein: 10g

Chia Coconut Porridge

Prep time: 5 minutes plus 30 minutes soaking | Cook time: 15 minutes | Serves 4

- ¾ cup water
- ¾ cup unsweetened almond milk
- 1 teaspoon pure vanilla extract
- ¼ cup chia seeds
- ¼ cup unsweetened shredded coconut
- 2 tablespoons raw honey
- ½ cup sliced fresh strawberries

1. In a medium bowl, whisk the water, almond milk, and vanilla until well blended.
2. Stir in the chia seeds, cover the bowl, and refrigerate it for a minimum of 30 minutes and up to overnight.
3. Stir the coconut and honey into the chilled porridge. Spoon the porridge into four bowls.
4. Serve topped with the strawberries.

PER SERVING

Calories: 124 | Total fat: 7g | Saturated Fat: 4g | Carbohydrates: 15g | Fiber: 4g | Protein: 2g

Lemon Almond Waffles

Prep time: 5 minutes | Cook time: 15 minutes | Serves 4

- 3 eggs
- 2/3 cup almond flour
- 2 ½ tsp baking powder
- A pinch of sea salt
- 1 ½ cups almond milk
- 2 tbsp olive oil
- 1 cup fresh almond butter
- 2 tbsp pure maple syrup
- 1 tsp fresh lemon juice

1. In a medium bowl, place the eggs, almond flour, baking powder, salt, and almond milk.
2. Mix until well combined.
3. Preheat a waffle iron and brush with some olive oil.
4. Pour in a quarter cup of the batter, close the iron and cook until the waffles are golden and crisp, 2-3 minutes.
5. Transfer the waffles to a plate and make more waffles until the ingredients are exhausted.
6. In a bowl, mix the almond butter with maple syrup and lemon juice.
7. Spread the top with the almond-lemon mixture and serve.

PER SERVING

Cal 430 | Fat 40g | Carbs 16.7g | Protein 7g

Creamy Sesame Bread

Prep time: 5 minutes | Cook time: 35 minutes | Serves 6

- 4 eggs
- 2/3 cup Greek yogurt
- 4 tbsp olive oil
- 1 cup coconut flour
- 2 tbsp psyllium husk powder
- 1 tsp sea salt
- 1 tsp baking powder
- 1 tbsp sesame seeds

1. Preheat your oven to 400°F.
2. Beat the eggs with yogurt and olive oil until well mixed.
3. Whisk in the coconut flour, psyllium husk powder, salt, and baking powder until adequately blended.
4. Grease a 9 x 5 inches baking tray with cooking spray, and spread the dough in the tray.
5. Allow the mixture to stand for 5 minutes and then brush with some sesame oil.
6. Sprinkle with the sesame seeds and bake the dough for 30 minutes until golden brown on top and set within.
7. Take out the bread and allow cooling for a few minutes.
8. Slice and serve.

PER SERVING

Cal 227 | Fat 15.3g | Carbs 15g | Protein 9g

Apple-Honey Smoothie

Prep time: 5 minutes | Cook time: 15 minutes | Serves 2

- 1 cup canned lite coconut milk
- 1 apple, cored and cut into chunks
- 1 banana
- ¼ cup almond butter
- 1 tablespoon raw honey
- ½ teaspoon ground cinnamon
- 4 ice cubes

1. In a blender, combine the coconut milk, apple, banana, almond butter, honey, and cinnamon. Blend until smooth.
2. Add the ice and blend until thick.

PER SERVING

Calories: 434 | Total fat: 30g | Saturated Fat: 26g | Carbohydrates: 46g | Fiber: 8g | Protein: 4g

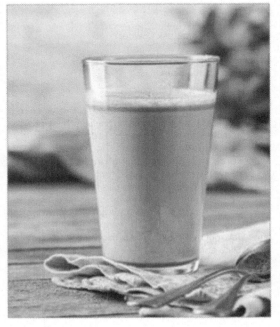

Sweet Potato Home Fries

Prep time: 15 minutes | Cook time: 6 to 8 hours | Serves 4 to 6

- 3 tablespoons extra-virgin olive oil, plus more for coating the slow cooker
- 2 pounds sweet potatoes, diced
- 1 red bell pepper, seeded and diced
- ½ medium onion, finely diced
- 1 teaspoon garlic powder
- 1 teaspoon sea salt
- 1 teaspoon dried rosemary, minced
- ½ teaspoon freshly ground black pepper

1. Coat the slow cooker with a thin layer of olive oil.
2. Put the sweet potatoes in the slow cooker, along with the red bell pepper and onion. Drizzle the olive oil as evenly as possible over the vegetables.
3. Sprinkle in the garlic powder, salt, rosemary, and pepper. Toss evenly to coat the sweet potatoes in the oil and seasonings.
4. Cover the cooker and set to low. Cook for 6 to 8 hours and serve.

PER SERVING

Calories: 296 | Total Fat: 11g | Total Carbs: 48g | Sugar: 10g | Fiber: 7g | Protein: 4g | Sodium: 705mg

German Chocolate Cake Protein Oats

Prep time: 15 minutes | Cook time: 6 to 8 hours | Serves 4 to 6

- 1 tablespoon coconut oil
- 2 cups rolled oats
- 2½ cups water
- 2 cups full-fat coconut milk
- ¼ cup unsweetened cacao powder
- 2 tablespoons collagen peptides (see Tip)
- ¼ teaspoon sea salt
- 2 tablespoons pecans
- 2 tablespoons unsweetened shredded coconut

1. Coat the slow cooker with the coconut oil.
2. In your slow cooker, combine the oats, water, coconut milk, cacao powder, collagen peptides, and salt. Stir to combine.
3. Cover the cooker and set to low. Cook for 6 to 8 hours.
4. Sprinkle the pecans and coconut on top and serve.

PER SERVING

Calories: 457 | Total Fat: 33g | Total Carbs: 36g | Sugar: 3g | Fiber: 7g | Protein: 10g | Sodium: 191mg

Sour Cream Coffee Cake with Browned Butter Glaze

Prep time: 15 minutes | Cook time: 45 minutes | Makes 1 Bundt cake

CAKE BATTER:

- 1 cup coconut flour, or 4 cups blanched almond flour
- 1 tablespoon ground cinnamon
- 2 teaspoons baking powder
- 1 teaspoon fine sea salt
- ¾ cup (1½ sticks) unsalted butter or coconut oil, softened
- 1½ cups Swerve confectioners'-style sweetener or equivalent amount of liquid or powdered sweetener
- 1½ teaspoons vanilla extract
- 8 large eggs (4 eggs if using almond flour)
- 1½ cups sour cream
- Cinnamon Filling:
- ½ cup Swerve confectioners'-style sweetener or equivalent amount of liquid or powdered sweetener
- 6 tablespoons (¾ stick) melted unsalted butter or coconut oil
- 1 tablespoon ground cinnamon
- 1 teaspoon vanilla extract
- Browned Butter Glaze:
- ¾ cup (1½ sticks) unsalted butter or coconut oil
- ¼ cup Swerve confectioners'-style sweetener or equivalent amount of liquid or powdered sweetener
- Cream Cheese Glaze:
- 1 (8-ounce) package cream cheese, softened
- ¼ cup unsweetened cashew milk
- ¼ cup Swerve confectioners'-style sweetener or equivalent amount of liquid or powdered sweetener
- Seeds scraped from 1 vanilla bean (about 8 inches long), or 1 teaspoon vanilla extract
- Chopped nuts of choice, for garnish (optional)

1. Preheat the oven to 350°F. Grease a 9-cup Bundt pan.
2. To make the cake batter, stir together the coconut flour, cinnamon, baking powder, and salt in a medium-sized bowl; set aside. In a large bowl, using a hand mixer, beat the softened butter, sweetener, and vanilla until light and fluffy. Add the eggs one at a time, beating for at least 1 minute after each addition. Beat in the flour mixture alternately with the sour cream. Pour half of the batter into the prepared pan.
3. To make the cinnamon filling, place the sweetener, melted butter, cinnamon, and vanilla in a small bowl and stir well to combine. Pour the filling evenly over the batter in the pan, using a knife to swirl it into the batter. Pour the rest of the batter into the pan.
4. Bake for 40 to 45 minutes, until a toothpick inserted in the center of the cake comes out clean. Let it cool in the pan for 10 minutes, then turn it out onto a wire rack to cool completely.
5. Meanwhile, make the browned butter glaze: Place the butter in a saucepan over medium-high heat and cook, whisking constantly, until brown (but not black!) flecks appear. Keep heating and whisking; the butter will froth up and then settle down. Remove the pan from the heat. (If using coconut oil, simply heat the oil in the pan until melted.) Add the sweetener and whisk until smooth. Set in the refrigerator to cool for 5 to 8 minutes.
6. Meanwhile, make the cream cheese glaze: Using the hand mixer, beat the softened cream cheese, cashew milk, and sweetener in a medium-sized bowl. Add the vanilla and stir well; taste and add more sweetener, if desired.

PER SERVING (1/12 OF THE CAKE)

Calories: 525 | Total Fat: 32g | Total Carbs: 56g | Sugar: 36g | Fiber: 0g | Protein: 7g | Sodium: 505mg

Bacon and Cheese Frittata

Prep time: 25 minutes | Cook time: 16 minutes | Serves 4

- 10 slices bacon
- 10 fresh eggs
- 3 tbsp butter, melted
- ½ cup almond milk
- Salt and black pepper to taste
- 1 ½ cups cheddar cheese, shredded
- ¼ cup chopped green onions

1. Preheat the oven to 400°F and grease a baking dish with cooking spray. Cook the bacon in a skillet over medium heat for 6 minutes. Once crispy, remove from the skillet to paper towels and discard grease. Chop into small pieces. Whisk the eggs, butter, milk, salt, and black pepper. Mix in the bacon and pour the mixture into the baking dish.
2. Sprinkle with cheddar cheese and green onions, and bake in the oven for 10 minutes or until the eggs are thoroughly cooked. Remove and cool the frittata for 3 minutes, slice into wedges, and serve warm with a dollop of Greek yogurt.

PER SERVING

Kcal: 325 | Fat: 28g | Net Carbs: 2g | Protein: 15g

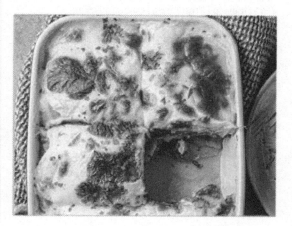

Tiramisu Muffins

Prep time: 10 minutes | Cook time: 20 minutes | Makes 12 muffins

MUFFINS:

- ½ cup coconut flour, or 2 cups blanched almond flour
- ½ cup Swerve confectioners'-style sweetener or equivalent amount of liquid or powdered sweetener
- 2 tablespoons unsweetened cocoa powder
- ¼ teaspoon fine sea salt
- ¼ teaspoon baking soda
- 6 large eggs (2 eggs if using almond flour), beaten
- 2 teaspoons rum extract
- Frosting:
- 1 (8-ounce) package mascarpone cheese (or Kite Hill brand cream cheese style spread if dairy-free), softened
- ¼ cup Swerve confectioners'-style sweetener or equivalent amount of liquid or powdered sweetener
- 1 ounce brewed decaf espresso or other strong brewed decaf coffee
- 1 teaspoon rum extract
- Unsweetened cocoa powder, for dusting

1. Preheat the oven to 350°F. Grease a standard-size 12-well muffin pan, or line the wells with paper liners.
2. In a medium-sized bowl, sift together the dry ingredients for the muffin batter. Slowly add the wet ingredients to the dry ingredients and stir until very smooth. Fill each well of the muffin pan about two-thirds full with the batter. Bake for 18 to 20 minutes, until a toothpick inserted in the center of a muffin comes out clean. Allow to cool in the pan before removing.
3. Meanwhile, make the frosting: Combine all the ingredients and mix until smooth. Set aside until the muffins are cool, then frost the muffins. Dust the frosted muffins with cocoa powder.
4. Store extras in an airtight container in the refrigerator for up to 1 week. The muffins can be frozen if unfrosted, but do not freeze the frosting.

PER SERVING (1 MUFFIN)

Calories: 497 | Total Fat: 31g | Total Carbs: 48g | Sugar: 31g | Fiber: 1g | Protein: 8g | Sodium: 209mg

Amazing Breakfast Sausage Bake

Prep time: 5 minutes | Cook time: 8 minutes | Serves 2

- ½ pound bulk pork sausage
- ½ teaspoon fine sea salt
- ⅓ cup beef bone broth, homemade or store-bought
- 2 strips bacon, diced
- ¼ cup shredded cheddar cheese
- ¼ cup thinly sliced green onions, for garnish

1. Preheat the broiler. Form the sausage into four 1½ by 2½-inch oval-shaped patties. Season on all sides with the salt.
2. Place the sausage patties in an 8-inch square casserole dish. Pour the broth over the patties and place the dish in the oven. Broil for 7 minutes or until the patties are cooked through.
3. Meanwhile, cook the diced bacon in a skillet over medium heat, stirring often, for 5 minutes or until the bacon is cooked through and crispy. Remove from the heat and set aside.
4. Remove the dish from the oven and top the sausage patties with the cheese and cooked bacon. Return the pan to the oven for 1 minute or until the cheese is melted. Garnish with the green onions.
5. Store extras in an airtight container in the refrigerator for up to 3 days. Reheat on a baking sheet in a preheated 350°F oven for 5 minutes or until warmed through.

PER SERVING

Calories: 319 | Total Fat: 20g | Total Carbs: 16g | Sugar: 3g | Fiber: 1g | Protein: 16g | Sodium: 384mg

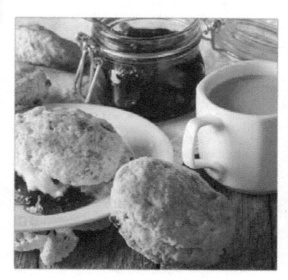

Monte Cristo Crepes

Prep time: 10 minutes (not including time to hard-boil eggs) | Cook time: 8 minutes | Serves 2

- Crepes:
- 2 large eggs
- 2 hard-boiled eggs
- 4 ounces cream cheese (½ cup) (Kite Hill brand cream cheese style spread if dairy-free), softened
- 1 tablespoon Swerve confectioners'-style sweetener or equivalent amount of liquid or powdered sweetener
- ½ teaspoon vanilla or almond extract
- Pinch of fine sea salt
- Coconut oil, for the pan
- Filling:
- 2 very thin slices ham
- 2 thin slices (1 ounce) Swiss cheese (omit for dairy-free)
- Raspberry glaze:
- 1½ ounces cream cheese (3 tablespoons) (Kite Hill brand cream cheese style spread if dairy-free), softened
- 2 tablespoons unsweetened cashew milk (or hemp milk if nut-free), warmed
- 2 tablespoons Swerve confectioners'-style sweetener or equivalent amount of liquid or powdered sweetener ½ teaspoon raspberry extract
- Special equipment:
- inch crepe pan or nonstick skillet

1. To make the crepe batter, place the raw eggs, hard-boiled eggs, cream cheese, sweetener, extract, and salt in a blender and blend until very smooth.
2. Grease an 8-inch crepe pan or nonstick skillet with coconut oil or coconut oil spray and set it over medium-high heat. When hot, pour ¼ cup of the batter into the skillet and swirl the skillet to spread the batter to the edges of the pan. Cook until golden brown, about 2 minutes, then flip and cook for another 2 minutes. Remove from the pan and repeat with the remaining batter.
3. Place 1 slice of ham and 1 slice of cheese in the center of each crepe. Fold the crepe in half, then fold it again into quarters.
4. Make the glaze: Place all the ingredients in a small bowl and whisk until well combined. Taste and add more sweetener and/or extract, if desired. Serve the crepes drizzled with the glaze.
5. Store extra crepes and glaze in separate airtight containers in the refrigerator for up to 3 days. Reheat the crepes on a baking sheet in a preheated 350°F oven for 5 minutes or until warmed through. Bring the glaze to room temperature, then drizzle it over the crepes.

PER SERVING (1 CREPE)

Calories: 138 | Total Fat: 6g | Total Carbs: 16g | Sugar: 7g | Fiber: 0g | Protein: 7g | Sodium: 144mg

Pumpkin Muffins

Prep time: 7 minutes | Cook time: 40 minutes | Makes 6 muffins

MUFFIN BATTER:

- 1½ cups blanched almond flour
- ½ teaspoon baking soda
- ¼ teaspoon fine sea salt
- 1 teaspoon ground cinnamon
- ½ teaspoon ground nutmeg
- ¼ teaspoon ground ginger
- ⅛ teaspoon ground cloves
- 2 tablespoons unsalted butter (or coconut oil if dairy-free), softened
- ½ cup Swerve confectioners'-style sweetener or equivalent amount of liquid or powdered sweetener
- 3 large eggs
- 1 cup fresh or canned pumpkin puree

CREAM CHEESE FILLING:

- 1 (8-ounce) package cream cheese (Kite Hill brand cream cheese style spread if dairy-free), softened
- ¼ cup Swerve confectioners'-style sweetener or equivalent amount of liquid or powdered sweetener
- 1 large egg yolk
- 2 teaspoons vanilla extract

1. Preheat the oven to 325°F. Grease or place paper liners in 6 wells of a standard-size muffin pan.
2. In a large mixing bowl, stir the almond flour, baking soda, salt, and spices until well combined. In another bowl, mix together the butter, sweetener, eggs, and pumpkin until smooth. Stir the wet ingredients into the dry. Spoon the batter into the prepared muffin cups, filling each about two-thirds full.
3. To make the filling, using a hand mixer, beat the cream cheese in a medium-sized bowl until smooth. Add the sweetener, egg yolk, and vanilla and beat until well combined. Top each muffin with about 1 tablespoon of the cream cheese filling and use a toothpick to swirl it into the batter.
4. Bake the muffins for 30 to 40 minutes, until a toothpick inserted into the center of a muffin comes out clean. Allow to cool before removing from the pan. Store extras in an airtight container in the refrigerator for up to 3 days. Reheat on a baking sheet in a preheated 350°F oven for 5 minutes or until warmed through.

PER SERVING (1 MUFFIN)

Calories: 195 | Total Fat: 9g | Total Carbs: 25g | Sugar: 12g | Fiber: 1g | Protein: 3g | Sodium: 195mg

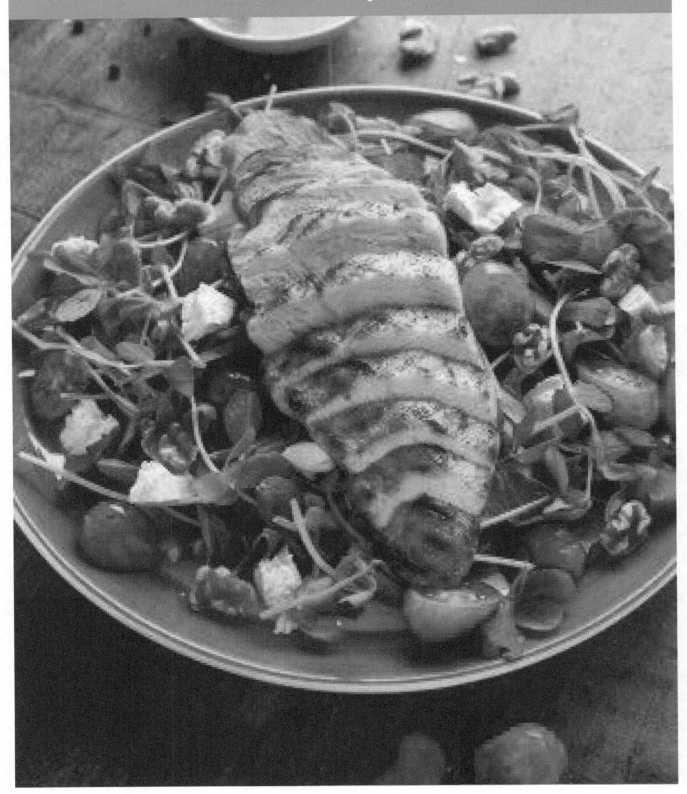

Chapter 5
Poultry

Chicken Bone Broth
Prep time: 15 minutes | Cook time: 6 to 8 hours | Serves 12

- 1 chicken carcass
- About 12 cups filtered water (enough to cover the bones)
- 2 carrots, roughly chopped
- 2 garlic cloves, roughly chopped
- 2 bay leaves
- 1 parsley sprig
- ¾ teaspoon sea salt
- ½ teaspoon dried oregano
- ½ teaspoon dried basil leaves
- 1 tablespoon apple cider vinegar

1. In your slow cooker, combine the chicken carcass, water, carrots, garlic, celery, onion, bay leaves, parsley, salt, oregano, basil, and vinegar.
2. Cover the cooker and set to low. Cook for 6 to 8 hours.
3. Skim off any scum from the surface of the broth, and pour the broth through a fine-mesh sieve into a large bowl, discarding the chicken and veggie scraps. Refrigerate the broth in an airtight container for up to 5 days, or freeze it for up to 3 months.

PER SERVING

Calories: 50 | Total Fat: 1g | Total Carbs: 1g | Sugar: 0g | Fiber: 0g | Protein: 9g | Sodium: 145mg

Coconut-Curry-Cashew Chicken
Prep time: 15 minutes | Cook time: 7 to 8 hours | Serves 4 to 6

- 1½ cups Chicken Bone Broth
- 1 (14-ounce) can full-fat coconut milk
- 1 teaspoon garlic powder
- 1 tablespoon red curry paste
- 1 teaspoon sea salt
- ½ teaspoon freshly ground black pepper
- ½ teaspoon coconut sugar
- 2 pounds boneless, skinless chicken breasts
- 1½ cup unsalted cashews
- ½ cup diced white onion

1. In a medium bowl, combine the broth, coconut milk, garlic powder, red curry paste, salt, pepper, and coconut sugar. Stir well.
2. Cover the cooker and set to low. Cook for 7 to 8 hours, or until the internal temperature of the chicken reaches 165°F on a meat thermometer and the juices run clear.
3. Shred the chicken with a fork, and mix it into the cooking liquid. You can also remove the chicken from the broth and chop it with a knife into bite-size pieces before returning it to the slow cooker. Serve.

PER SERVING

Calories: 714 | Total Fat: 43g | Total Carbs: 21g | Sugar: 5g | Fiber: 3g | Protein: 57g | Sodium: 1,606mg

Easy Chicken Chili
Prep time: 30 minutes | Cook time: 15 minutes | Serves 4

- 4 chicken breasts, skinless, boneless, cubed
- tbsp butter
- ½ onion, chopped
- cups chicken broth
- 8 oz diced tomatoes
- 2 oz tomato puree
- 1 tbsp chili powder
- 1 tbsp cumin
- ½ tbsp garlic powder
- 1 serrano pepper, minced
- ½ cup shredded cheddar cheese
- Salt and black pepper to taste

1. Set a large pan over medium-high heat and add the chicken. Cover with water and bring to a boil. Cook until no longer pink, for 10 minutes. Transfer the chicken to a flat surface to shred with forks.
2. In a large pot, pour in the butter and set over medium heat. Sauté onion until transparent for 5 minutes. Stir in the chicken, tomatoes, cumin, serrano pepper, garlic powder, tomato puree, broth, and chili powder. Adjust the seasoning and let the mixture boil. Reduce heat to simmer for about 10 minutes. Divide chili among bowls and top with shredded cheese to serve.

PER SERVING

Kcal: 421 | Fat: 21g | Net Carbs: 5.6g | Protein: 45g

Chicken Stir-Fry
Prep time: 15 minutes | Cook time: 15 minutes | Serves 4

- 3 tablespoons extra-virgin olive oil
- 6 scallions, white and green parts, chopped
- 1 cup broccoli florets
- 1 pound boneless, skinless chicken breasts, cut into bite-size pieces
- 1 recipe stir-fry sauce
- Tablespoons toasted sesame seeds (optional)

1. In a large nonstick skillet over medium-high heat, heat the olive oil until it shimmers.
2. Add the scallions, broccoli, and chicken. Cook for 5 to 7 minutes, stirring occasionally, until the chicken is cooked and the vegetables are tender.
3. Add the stir-fry sauce. Cook for 5 minutes, stirring, until the sauce reduces.
4. Garnish with sesame seeds, if using.

PER SERVING

Calories: 363 | Total Fat: 22g | Total Carbs: 7g | Sugar: 2g | Fiber: 2g | Protein: 36g | Sodium: 993mg

Spanish Chicken

Prep time: 60 minutes | Cook time: 30 minutes | Serves 4

- 1/2 cup mushrooms, chopped
- pound chorizo sausages, chopped
- tbsp avocado oil
- 4 cherry peppers, chopped
- 1 red bell pepper, seeded, chopped
- onion, peeled and sliced
- tbsp garlic, minced
- 2 cups tomatoes, chopped
- 4 chicken thighs
- Salt and black pepper, to taste
- ½ cup chicken stock
- 1 tsp turmeric
- tbsp vinegar
- tsp dried oregano
- Fresh parsley, chopped, for serving

1. Set a pan over medium heat and warm half of the avocado oil, stir in the chorizo sausages, and cook for 5-6 minutes until browned; remove to a bowl. Heat the rest of the oil, place in the chicken thighs, and apply pepper and salt for seasoning. Cook each side for 3 minutes and set aside on a bowl.
2. In the same pan, add the onion, bell pepper, cherry peppers, and mushrooms, and cook for 4 minutes. Stir in the garlic and cook for 2 minutes. Pour in the stock, turmeric, salt, tomatoes, pepper, vinegar, and oregano. Stir in the chorizo sausages and chicken, place everything to the oven at 400°F, and bake for 30 minutes. Ladle into serving bowls and garnish with chopped parsley to serve.

PER SERVING

Kcal: 415 | Fat: 33g | Net Carbs: 4g | Protein: 25g

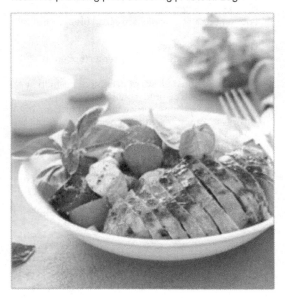

Chicken Salad Sandwiches

Prep time: 10 minutes | Cook time: 15 minutes | Serves 4

- 2 cups chopped, cooked, skinless chicken from a rotisserie chicken
- ¼ cup anti-inflammatory mayonnaise (here)
- 1 red bell pepper, minced
- 2 tablespoons chopped fresh tarragon leaves
- 2 teaspoons dijon mustard
- ½ teaspoon sea salt
- 8 slices whole-wheat bread

1. In a medium bowl, stir together the chicken, mayonnaise, red bell pepper, tarragon, mustard, and salt.
2. Spread on 4 slices of bread and top with the remaining bread.

PER SERVING

Calories: 315 | Total Fat: 9g | Total Carbs: 30g | Sugar: 6g | Fiber: 4g | Protein: 28g | Sodium: 677mg

Easy Chicken and Broccoli

Prep time: 10 minutes | Cook time: 7 minutes | Serves 4

- 3 tablespoons extra-virgin olive oil
- 1½ pounds boneless, skinless chicken breasts, cut into bite-size pieces
- 1½ cups broccoli florets, or chopped broccoli stems
- ½ onion, chopped
- ½ teaspoon sea salt
- ¼ teaspoon freshly ground black pepper
- 3 garlic cloves, minced
- 2 cups cooked brown rice

1. In a large nonstick skillet over medium-high heat, heat the olive oil until it shimmers.
2. Add the chicken, broccoli, onion, salt, and pepper. Cook for about 7 minutes, stirring occasionally, until the chicken is cooked.
3. Add the garlic. Cook for 30 seconds, stirring constantly.
4. Toss with the brown rice to serve.

PER SERVING

Calories: 345 | Total Fat: 14g | Total Carbs: 41g | Sugar: 1g | Fiber: 3g | Protein: 14g | Sodium: 276mg

Rosemary Chicken

Prep time: 10 minutes | Cook time: 20 minutes | Serves 4

- 1½ pounds chicken breast tenders
- 2 tablespoons extra-virgin olive oil
- 2 tablespoons chopped fresh rosemary leaves
- ½ teaspoon sea salt
- ⅛ teaspoon freshly ground black pepper

1. Preheat the oven to 425°f.
2. Place the chicken tenders on a rimmed baking sheet. Brush them with the olive oil and sprinkle with the rosemary, salt, and pepper.
3. Bake for 15 to 20 minutes, or until the juices run clear.

PER SERVING

Calories: 389 | Total Fat: 20g | Total Carbs: 1g | Sugar: 0g | Fiber: <1g | Protein: 49g | Sodium: 381mg

Thyme Chicken Thighs

Prep time: 30 minutes | Cook time: 8 minutes | Serves 4

- ½ cup chicken stock
- 1 tbsp olive oil
- ½ cup chopped onion
- 4 chicken thighs
- ¼ cup heavy cream
- 2 tbsp Dijon mustard
- 1 tsp thyme
- 1 tsp garlic powder

1. Heat the olive oil in a pan. Cook the chicken for about 4 minutes per side. Set aside. Sauté the onion in the same pan for 3 minutes, add the stock, and simmer for 5 minutes. Stir in mustard and heavy cream, along with thyme and garlic powder.
2. Pour the sauce over the chicken and serve.

PER SERVING

Kcal: 528 | Fat: 42g | Net Carbs: 4g | Protein: 33g

Leftover Chicken Salad Sandwiches

Prep time: 5 minutes | Cook time: 5 minutes | Serves 4

- 2 cups leftover cooked, skinless chicken, pulled
- 1 spring onion, finely sliced
- ¼ cup paleo mayonnaise
- 1 red bell pepper, sliced
- 2 tbsp chopped tarragon
- 2 tsp Dijon mustard
- ½ tsp sea salt
- 8 slices whole-wheat bread

1. Combine chicken, mayonnaise, red bell pepper, tarragon, mustard, spring onion, and salt in a bowl.
2. To make the sandwiches, spread one side of 4 bread slices with the mixture and top with the remaining bread.
3. Serve.

PER SERVING

Cal 320| Fat 10g| Carbs 31g| Protein 4g

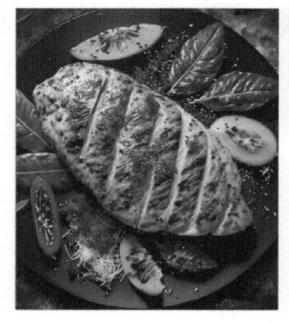

Grilled Chicken Sandwiches

Prep time: 5 minutes | Cook time: 15 minutes | Serves 4

- 2 tbsp olive oil
- 4 chicken breast halves
- Sea salt and pepper to taste
- 6 roasted red pepper slices
- 1 tbsp Dijon mustard
- ¼ cup paleo mayonnaise
- 4 whole-wheat buns, halved

1. Pound the chicken with a rolling pin to ½-inch thickness.
2. Preheat your grill to medium-high heat.
3. Sprinkle the chicken breasts with salt and pepper and brush them with olive oil.
4. Place them on the hot grill and cook for 8 minutes on all sides until cooked through.
5. In the meantime, place the mustard, mayonnaise, and 2 red pepper slices in a food processor and pulse until smooth.
6. To make the sandwiches, cover the bottom halves of the buns with the mayo mixture, followed by the remaining roasted pepper slices and chicken.
7. Finish with the top bun halves.
8. Serve immediately.

PER SERVING

Cal 320| Fat 16g| Carbs 37g| Protein 7g

Chicken Skewers with Celery Fries

Prep time: 60 minutes | Cook time: 40 minutes | Serves 4

- 2 chicken breasts
- ½ tsp salt
- 2 tbsp olive oil
- 1/4 cup chicken broth
- For The Fries
- 1 lb celery root
- 2 tbsp olive oil
- ½ tsp salt
- ¼ tsp ground black pepper

1. Set oven to 400°F. Grease and line a baking sheet. In a bowl, mix oil, spices and the chicken; set in the fridge for 10 minutes while covered. Peel and chop celery root to form fry shapes and place into a separate bowl. Apply oil to coat and add pepper and salt for seasoning. Arrange to the baking tray in an even layer and bake for 10 minutes.
2. Take the chicken from the refrigerator and thread onto the skewers. Place over the celery, pour in the chicken broth, then set in the oven for 30 minutes. Serve with lemon wedges.

PER SERVING

Kcal: 579 | Fat: 43g | Net Carbs: 6g | Protein: 39

Chicken Stir-Fry with Bell Pepper

Prep time: 5 minutes | Cook time: 25 minutes | Serves 4

- 3 tbsp avocado oil
- ½ tsp red pepper flakes
- 1 red bell pepper, chopped
- 1 onion, chopped
- 1 ½ lb chicken breasts, cubed
- 2 garlic cloves, minced
- Sea salt and pepper to taste

1. Warm the avocado oil in a skillet over medium heat and place in bell pepper, onion, and chicken.
2. Sauté for 10 minutes.
3. Stir in garlic, salt, and pepper and cook for another 30 seconds.
4. Sprinkle with red flakes and serve.

PER SERVING

Cal 180| Fat 14g| Carbs 7g| Protein 2g

Chicken Breasts in Adobo Sauce

Prep time: 5 minutes | Cook time: 20 minutes | Serves 4

- 1 tbsp Adobo seasoning
- 3 tbsp olive oil
- 1 ½ lb chicken breast strips
- 2 tsp ground turmeric
- 3 tsp low-sodium soy sauce
- 1 tsp garlic powder
- 1 tsp onion powder

1. Rub the chicken with adobo seasoning, garlic powder, onion powder, and turmeric.
2. Warm the olive oil in a skillet over medium heat and place in chicken.
3. Cook for 7-10 minutes until the chicken is thoroughly cooked.
4. Stir in the soy sauce for 3 minutes.
5. Serve immediately.

PER SERVING

Cal 700| Fat 53g| Carbs 12g| Protein 2g

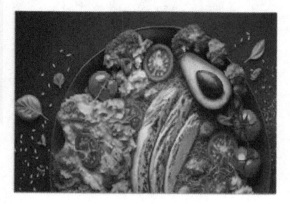

Cheesy Chicken Bake with Zucchini

Prep time: 45 minutes | Cook time: 30 minutes | Serves 6

- 2 lb chicken breasts, cubed
- 1 tbsp butter
- 1 cup green bell peppers, sliced
- 1 cup yellow onions, sliced
- zucchini, cubed
- garlic cloves, divided
- 2 tsp Italian seasoning
- ½ tsp salt
- ½ tsp black pepper
- 8 oz cream cheese, softened
- ½ cup mayonnaise
- 2 tbsp Worcestershire sauce (sugar-free)
- 2 cups cheddar cheese, shredded

1. Set oven to 370°F and grease and line a baking dish.
2. Set a pan over medium heat. Place in the butter and let melt, then add in the chicken. Cook until lightly browned, about 5 minutes. Place in onions, zucchini, black pepper, garlic, bell peppers, salt, and 1 tsp of Italian seasoning. Cook until tender and set aside.
3. In a bowl, mix cream cheese, garlic, remaining seasoning, mayonnaise, and Worcestershire sauce. Stir in meat and sauteed vegetables. Place the mixture into the prepared baking dish, sprinkle with the shredded cheddar cheese and insert into the oven. Cook until browned for 30 minutes.

PER SERVING

Kcal: 489 | Fat: 37g | Net Carbs: 4.5g | Protein: 21g

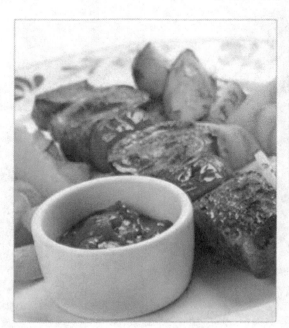

One Pot Chicken with Mushrooms

Prep time: 35 minutes | Cook time: 20 minutes | Serves 6

- 2 cups sliced mushrooms
- ½ tsp onion powder
- ½ tsp garlic powder
- ¼ cup butter
- 1 tsp Dijon mustard
- 1 tbsp tarragon, chopped
- 1 pounds chicken thighs
- Salt and black pepper, to taste

1. Season the thighs with salt, pepper, garlic, and onion powder. Melt the butter in a skillet, and cook the chicken until browned; set aside. Add mushrooms to the same fat and cook for about 5 minutes.
2. Stir in Dijon mustard and ½ cup of water. Return the chicken to the skillet. Season to taste with salt and pepper, reduce the heat and cover, and let simmer for 15 minutes. Stir in tarragon. Serve warm.

PER SERVING

Kcal: 447 | Fat: 37g | Net Carbs: 1g | Protein: 31g

Chicken in Creamy Tomato Sauce

Prep time: 20 minutes | Cook time: 5 minutes | Serves 6

- 2 tbsp butter
- 6 chicken thighs
- Pink salt and black pepper to taste
- 14 oz canned tomato sauce
- 2 tsp Italian seasoning
- ½ cup heavy cream
- 1 cup shredded Parmesan cheese Parmesan cheese to garnish.

1. In a saucepan, melt the butter over medium heat, season the chicken with salt and black pepper, and cook for 5 minutes on each side to brown. Plate the chicken.
2. Pour the tomato sauce and Italian seasoning in the pan and cook covered for 8 minutes. Adjust the taste with salt and black pepper and stir in the heavy cream and Parmesan cheese.
3. Once the cheese has melted, return the chicken to the pot, and simmer for 4 minutes. Dish the chicken with sauce, garnish with more Parmesan cheese, and serve with zoodles.

PER SERVING

Kcal: 456 | Fat: 38.2g | Net Carbs: 2g | Protein: 24g

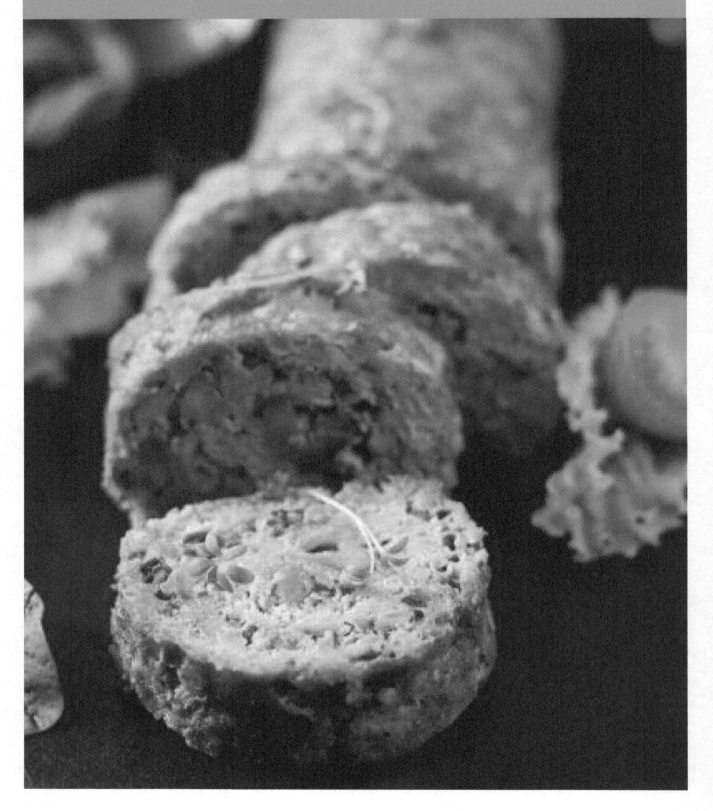

Chapter 6
Meat

Sausage & White Bean Soup

Prep time: 15 minutes | Cook time: 6 to 7 hours | Serves 4 to 6

- 1 pound pre-cooked pork sausage, thinly sliced into coins
- 2 (15-ounce) cans cannellini beans, rinsed and drained well
- 5 carrots, diced
- 1 medium onion, diced
- 1 celery stalk, minced
- 2 bay leaves
- 1 teaspoon garlic powder
- ½ teaspoon dried oregano
- ½ teaspoon dried basil leaves
- 6 cups broth of choice
- 4 cups shredded, de-ribbed kale

1. In your slow cooker, combine the sausage, beans, carrots, onion, celery, bay leaves, garlic powder, oregano, basil, broth, and kale.
2. Cover the cooker and set to low. Cook for 6 to 7 hours.
3. Remove and discard the bay leaves before serving.

PER SERVING

Calories: 712 | Total Fat: 36g | Total Carbs: 52g | Sugar: 9g | Fiber: 13g | Protein: 47g | Sodium: 1,926mg

Filet Mignons Florentine

Prep time: 5 minutes (not including time to make hollandaise) | Cook time: 10 minutes | Serves 2

- 1 tablespoon keto fat, for frying
- 2 (3-ounce) filet mignons, about 1¼ inches thick
- 1½ teaspoons fine sea salt
- ½ teaspoon ground black pepper
- 1 large tomato, thinly sliced
- 2 tablespoons minced shallots
- 2 cups fresh spinach
- ¼ cup Easy Basil Hollandaise

1. Heat a cast-iron skillet over medium-high heat, then put the fat in the pan. While the skillet is heating, pat the steaks dry with a paper towel and season well with the salt and pepper. Place the steaks in the hot fat and sear on one side for 3 minutes, then flip and sear on the other side for 3 minutes or until done to your liking. (A total of 6 minutes' cooking time will give you medium-rare steaks.) Set the steaks on a cutting board to rest for 10 minutes while you prepare the rest of the meal.
2. Place 3 slices of tomato on each plate. Place the shallots in the skillet in which you cooked the steaks and sauté over medium-high heat for 2 minutes. Add the spinach and sauté for another 2 minutes or until wilted. Season to taste with salt. Top the tomatoes with the wilted greens.
3. Place a rested steak on top of the greens, then drizzle 2 tablespoons of the hollandaise over each steak.

4. This dish is best served fresh, but any extras can be stored in an airtight container in the refrigerator for up to 3 days. Reheat the steak on a baking sheet in a preheated 350°F oven for 5 minutes or until warmed through. To reheat the hollandaise, see .

PER SERVING

Calories: 640 | Total fat: 47g | Saturated fat: 20g | Cholesterol: 245mg | Sodium: 630mg | Total carbohydrates: 6g | Dietary fiber: 2g | Sugars: 3g | Protein: 49g

Steak with Blue Cheese Whip

Prep time: 5 minutes | Cook time: about 10 minutes | Serves 2

- 1 (12-ounce) T-bone steak, about ¾ inch thick
- 1¼ teaspoons fine sea salt
- ½ teaspoon ground black pepper
- 1 tablespoon keto fat, for frying
- Blue Cheese Whip:
- ¼ cup heavy cream
- ¼ ounce blue cheese, finely crumbled
- ⅛ teaspoon fine sea salt

1. Preheat the oven to 400°F.
2. Season the steak generously on all sides with the salt and pepper. Heat a cast-iron skillet over medium-high heat, then melt the fat in the pan. When hot, sear the steak for 3 minutes on each side.
3. Place the skillet in the oven to cook the steak to your desired doneness, using a meat thermometer to determine the internal temperature (see chart below). Remove the skillet from the heat and allow the steak to rest for 10 minutes before slicing and serving.
4. While the steak is resting, make the blue cheese whip: Place the cream in a stand mixer and mix until stiff peaks form. Stir in the blue cheese and salt until well blended. (The whip can be made ahead and stored in an airtight container in the refrigerator for up to 3 days.)
5. Serve each portion of steak with 2 tablespoons of the blue cheese whip.
6. This dish is best served fresh, but any extras can be stored in an airtight container in the refrigerator for up to 3 days. Reheat on a rimmed baking sheet in a preheated 350°F oven for 5 minutes or until warmed through.

PER SERVING

Calories: 620 | Total fat: 48g | Saturated fat: 24g | Cholesterol: 190mg | Sodium: 630mg | Total carbohydrates: 1g | Dietary fiber: 0g | Sugars: 1g | Protein: 45g

Ham 'n' Grits with Redeye Gravy

Prep time: 8 minutes (not including time to make grits) |
Cook time: 20 minutes | Serves 2

- 2 tablespoons ghee or unsalted butter, plus extra for serving
- 2 (½-inch-thick) ham steaks (about 1½ pounds total), cut into ½-inch cubes
- ¼ cup diced onions
- ½ cup brewed decaf coffee, or 1 shot decaf espresso diluted with ¼ cup water
- 1 batch Keto Grits, for serving
- Sliced green onions, for garnish

1. Melt the ghee in a large cast-iron skillet over medium-high heat. Place the ham and onions in the pan and cook, stirring often, for 6 minutes or until the cubes of ham are brown and crispy. Remove the ham to a warm serving plate.
2. Pour the coffee into the skillet with the onions and, using a whisk, scrape up any browned bits from the bottom of the skillet. Cook for 10 minutes or until the gravy has reduced a bit and thickened.
3. Place the keto grits on a serving platter. Top them with the ham and gravy and garnish with green onions. Store extras in an airtight container in the refrigerator for up to 3 days. Reheat in a baking dish in a preheated 350°F oven for 5 minutes or until warmed through.

PER SERVING

Calories: 540 | Total fat: 23g | Saturated fat: 8g | Cholesterol: 70mg | Sodium: 1200mg | Total carbohydrates: 60g | Dietary fiber: 2g | Sugars: 1g | Protein: 24g

Traditional Beef Bolognese

Prep time: 5 minutes | Cook time: 8 hours 10 minutes | Serves 4

- 3 garlic cloves, minced
- 1 tbsp extra-virgin olive oil
- 1 chopped onion
- 1 chopped celery stalk
- 1 chopped carrot
- 1 lb ground beef
- 1 can diced tomatoes
- 1 tbsp white wine vinegar
- ⅛ tsp ground nutmeg
- ½ cup red wine
- ½ tsp red pepper flakes
- Sea salt and pepper to taste

1. Grease your slow cooker with olive oil.
2. Add onion, garlic, celery, carrot, ground beef, tomatoes, vinegar, nutmeg, wine, pepper flakes, salt, and pepper.
3. Using a fork, break up the ground beef as much as possible.
4. Cover the cooker and cook for 8 hours on "Low".
5. Serve and enjoy!

PER SERVING

Cal 315| Fat 20g| Carbs 10g| Protein 21g

Meatballs with Brown Gravy

Prep time: 5 minutes | Cook time: 35 minutes | Serves 4

MEATBALLS:

- 1 tablespoon coconut oil (or unsalted butter if not dairy-sensitive)
- ¼ cup chopped onions
- 1 teaspoon fine sea salt
- 2 pounds ground beef
- 1 cup finely chopped mushrooms
- 1 cup grated Parmesan cheese (omit for dairy-free)
- 1 large egg
- Gravy:
- 2 tablespoons bacon fat or lard (or unsalted butter if not dairy-sensitive)
- 1 cup beef bone broth, homemade or store-bought
- 1 teaspoon coconut aminos or wheat-free tamari
- ¼ teaspoon fine sea salt
- ¼ teaspoon ground black pepper
- 1 teaspoon fish sauce (optional, for umami flavor)

1. Preheat the oven to 350°F.
2. Heat the coconut oil in a heavy-bottomed skillet. Add the onions, sprinkle with the salt, and cook gently for about 5 minutes, until the onions are translucent. Remove the onions to a bowl to cool.
3. Put the ground beef, mushrooms, Parmesan cheese, and egg in a bowl. When the onion mixture is no longer hot to the touch, add it to the meat mixture and work everything together with your hands.
4. Shape the meat mixture into 2-inch balls and place the balls on a rimmed baking sheet. Bake for 30 minutes or until the meatballs are cooked through.
5. To make the gravy, place all the ingredients for the gravy in a saucepan. Boil, stirring often, for 10 minutes or until the gravy is thick and bubbly. Serve the meatballs with the gravy.
6. Store extras in an airtight container in the refrigerator for up to 3 days. Reheat in a baking dish in a preheated 350°F oven for 5 minutes or until warmed through.

PER SERVING

Calories: 390 | Total fat: 29g | Saturated fat: 11g | Cholesterol: 110mg | Sodium: 840mg | Total carbohydrates: 9g | Dietary fiber: 0g | Sugars: 1g | Protein: 22g

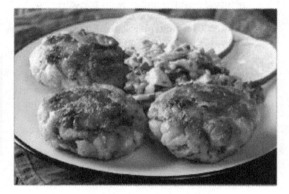

Pork and Cheddar Sausages

Prep time: 20 minutes, plus 3 to 4 hours to chill meat, soak casings, and rest sausage | Cook time: 10 minutes | Makes 12 sausages

- 2½ pounds pork butt
- ½ pound pork fat
- ½ cup coconut vinegar
- 6 feet medium hog casings
- ⅓ cup ice-cold beef or chicken bone broth, homemade or store-bought
- 2 cups finely diced sharp cheddar cheese
- ¼ cup chopped green onions or 2 tablespoons dried chives
- Cloves squeezed from 1 head roasted garlic, or 2 cloves raw garlic, smashed to paste
- 1 tablespoon fine sea salt
- 1 tablespoon lard or coconut oil, for the pan
- Keto dipping sauce(s) of choice, such as stone-ground mustard, for serving (optional)

1. Line a rimmed baking sheet with parchment paper. Cut the pork butt and fat into 1-inch cubes and spread them out on the lined baking sheet. Freeze for 1 hour.
2. After the meat and fat have been in the freezer for 30 minutes, fill a large bowl with the coconut vinegar and 2 quarts of water. Place the casings in the liquid to soak for 30 minutes.
3. Remove the pork meat and fat from the freezer and grind it using the coarse disk of a meat grinder (I use my KitchenAid food grinder attachment). In a large bowl, place the ground pork butt and fat, broth, cheese, green onions, garlic, and salt; combine well using your hands. Cook up a small dab of the sausage mixture in a skillet over medium heat; taste the cooked sausage and add more salt to the raw sausage mixture, if desired. Place the bowl of sausage in the freezer for 30 minutes to chill and firm up before stuffing the casings.
4. Load a sausage stuffer (I use my KitchenAid sausage stuffer attachment) with the presoaked casings and stuff the casings by pushing the sausage mixture through the attachment. Twist the sausages into links about 5 inches in length. (If you do not have a sausage stuffer, you can form the sausage mixture into 12 large patties instead.) Refrigerate the sausages for a few hours to allow the flavors to meld. Cook them within 3 days.
5. To cook the sausages, melt 1 tablespoon of lard or coconut oil in a large skillet over medium heat. Poke a few small holes in each sausage link. Sauté the sausages for 10 minutes or until their internal temperature reaches 160°F. Serve with keto dipping sauce, if desired. Once cooked, the sausages will keep in an airtight container in the refrigerator for up to 5 days. They can also be frozen for up to a month.

PER SERVING

Calories: 315|Total fat: 26g|Saturated fat: 9g| Cholesterol: 65mg| Sodium: 725mg| Protein: 18g| Fiber: 9g

Lettuce-Wrapped Beef Roast

Prep time: 5 minutes | Cook time: 8 hours 10 minutes | Serves 4

- 2 lb beef chuck roast
- 1 shallot, diced
- 1 cup beef broth
- 3 tbsp coconut aminos
- 1 tbsp rice vinegar
- 1 tsp garlic powder
- 1 tsp olive oil
- ½ tsp ground ginger
- ¼ tsp red pepper flakes
- 8 romaine lettuce leaves
- 1 tbsp sesame seeds
- 1 scallion, diced

1. Place the beef, shallot, broth, coconut aminos, vinegar, garlic powder, olive oil, ginger, and red pepper flakes in your slow cooker.
2. Cover the cooker and set to "Low".
3. Cook for 8 hours.
4. Scoop spoonfuls of the beef mixture into each lettuce leaf.
5. Top with sesame seeds and scallion.

PER SERVING

Cal 425| Fat 22g| Carbs 12g| Protein 45g

Tangy Beef Carnitas

Prep time: 5 minutes | Cook time: 25 minutes | Serves 4

- 1 tsp cayenne pepper
- 1 tsp paprika
- ¼ cup fresh cilantro leaves
- 6 tbsp olive oil
- 4 garlic cloves, minced
- 1 jalapeño pepper, chopped
- 1½ lb beef flank steak
- Sea salt and pepper to taste
- 1 cup guacamole

1. Place cilantro, 4 tbsp of olive oil, garlic, cayenne pepper, paprika, and jalapeño in your food processor and pulse until it reaches a paste consistency.
2. Reserve 1 tbsp of the paste.
3. Rub the flank steak with the remaining paste.
4. Warm the remaining olive oil in a skillet over medium heat.
5. Sear the steak for 15 minutes on all sides until browned.
6. Remove the meat to a cutting board and let it cool for 5 minutes.
7. Cut it against the grain into ½-inch-thick slices.
8. Put the beef in a bowl and add the reserved garlic paste| toss to combine.
9. Serve with guacamole.

PER SERVING

Cal 720| Fat 53g| Carbs 13g| Protein 2g

Beef Bone Broth

Prep time: 15 minutes | Cook time: 18 to 24 hours | Serves 4

- 2 pounds beef marrow bones
- 2 cups roughly chopped onions, celery, carrots, garlic, or scraps (a combination based on what's on hand or what you've saved)
- 2 bay leaves
- 1 tablespoon apple cider vinegar
- Filtered water, to cover the ingredients

1. In your slow cooker, combine the bones, onion, celery, carrots, garlic, bay leaves, and vinegar. Add enough water to cover the ingredients.
2. Cover the cooker and set to low. Cook for 18 to 24 hours. The longer it cooks, the more nutrients you get from the bones and vegetables.
3. Skim off and discard any foam from the surface. Ladle the broth through a fine-mesh sieve or cheesecloth into a large bowl. Transfer to airtight containers to store.
4. Keep refrigerated for 3 to 4 days. Freeze any excess for up to 3 months.

PER SERVING

Calories: 50 | Total Fat: 1g | Total Carbs: 2g | Sugar: 0g | Fiber: 0g | Protein: 6g | Sodium: 220mg

Hot & Spicy Beef Chili

Prep time: 5 minutes | Cook time: 20 minutes | Serves 4

- 2 tbsp olive oil
- 1 tsp dried Mexican oregano
- 1 lb ground beef
- 1 onion, chopped
- 2 (28-oz) cans diced tomatoes
- 2 (14-oz) cans kidney beans,
- 1 tbsp red chili powder
- 1 tsp garlic powder
- ½ tsp sea salt

1. Warm the olive oil in a heavy-bottomed pot over medium heat.
2. Then, brown the ground beef for 5 minutes, crumbling with a wide spatula.
3. Mix in tomatoes, Mexican oregano, kidney beans, red chili powder, garlic powder, and salt and bring to a simmer.
4. Let it cook, partially covered, for 10 minutes longer.
5. Serve warm.

PER SERVING

Cal 900| Fat 21g| Carbs 64g| Protein 18g

Stir fried Beef with Vegetables

Prep time: 5 minutes | Cook time: 15 minutes | Serves 4

- 1 lb flank steak, sliced into strips
- 4 tsp reduced-salt soy sauce
- 2 tbsp olive oil
- 1 cup broccoli florets
- 1 cup green beans, chopped
- 1 zucchini, chopped

1. Warm the olive oil in a skillet over medium heat.
2. Brown beef strips for 5-7 minutes, stirring occasionally.
3. Set aside.
4. Place the broccoli, green beans, and zucchini in the skillet and cook for 5 minutes until they're crisp-tender.
5. Put the beef back in the pot and pour in the soy sauce.
6. Cook for another 3 minutes.
7. Serve immediately.

PER SERVING

Cal 300| Fat 18g| Carbs 5g| Protein 2g

Rosemary Lamb Chops

Prep time: 5 minutes | Cook time: 45 minutes | Serves 4

- 4 garlic cloves, mashed
- 8 lamb chops
- 2 tbsp chopped rosemary
- ¼ cup extra-virgin olive oil
- 1 tsp Dijon mustard
- Sea salt and pepper to taste

1. Mix the olive oil, rosemary, garlic, Dijon mustard, salt, and pepper in a bowl.
2. Add the lamb chops and toss to coat R.
3. Cover the dish with plastic wrap and marinate the chops at room temperature for 30 minutes.
4. Preheat your oven to 425°F.
5. Bake the lamb chops for 15-20 minutes, or until they are sizzling and browned.
6. Serve.

PER SERVING

Cal 645| Fat 33g| Carbs 3g| Protein 79g

Bangers and Mash with Onion Gravy

Prep time: 8 minutes (not including time to make fauxtatoes) | Cook time: 20 minutes | Serves 4

- 4 (4-ounce) banger sausages
- Onion Gravy:
- 2 tablespoons unsalted butter
- 1 cup sliced onions
- 2 cups beef bone broth, homemade or store-bought
- 1 teaspoon chopped fresh thyme or other herb of choice
- Fine sea salt and ground black pepper
- 1 batch Mashed Fauxtatoes, for serving

1. Preheat a grill or broiler to high heat.
2. Bring a pot of water to a boil. Add the sausages and boil for 8 minutes.
3. Meanwhile, make the onion gravy: Melt the butter in a skillet over medium-high heat. Add the onions and cook until translucent and just starting to brown, about 6 minutes. Add the broth and increase the heat to a boil. Boil for 10 minutes or until the liquid is reduced by half. Add the thyme and season with salt and pepper.
4. Place the boiled sausages on the grill or, if using the oven broiler, on a rimmed baking sheet and grill or broil for 1 to 2 minutes, until the outsides are charred to your liking.
5. To serve, place ½ cup of mashed fauxtatoes on each plate. Top with a sausage and cover with the onion gravy.
6. Store extras in an airtight container in the refrigerator for up to 3 days. Reheat the sausages on a rimmed baking sheet in a preheated 350°F oven for 5 minutes or until warmed through. Reheat the gravy in a small saucepan over medium heat until warmed.

Saucy Tomato Beef Meatballs

Prep time: 5 minutes | Cook time: 8 hours 10 minutes | Serves 6

- 1 ½ lb ground beef
- 1 can crushed tomatoes
- 1 large egg
- 1 small onion, minced
- ¼ cup minced mushrooms
- 1 tsp garlic powder
- Sea salt and pepper to taste
- ½ tsp dried thyme
- ¼ tsp ground ginger
- ¼ tsp red pepper flakes

1. Combine the ground beef, egg, onion, mushrooms, garlic powder, salt, pepper, thyme, ginger, and red pepper flakes in a large bowl.
2. Mix well.
3. Form the beef mixture into about 12 meatballs.
4. Pour the tomatoes into your slow cooker.
5. Gently arrange the meatballs on top.
6. Cover the cooker and set to "Low".
7. Cook for 8 hours.

PER SERVING

Cal 130| Fat 9g| Carbs 2g| Protein 10g

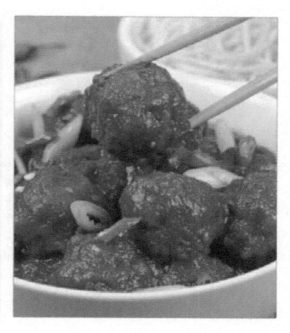

Mustardy Leg of Lamb

Prep time: 5 minutes | Cook time: 6 hours 10 minutes | Serves 4

- 1 (3-lb) lamb leg
- ½ cup white wine
- 1½ cups chicken broth
- 1 onion, roughly chopped
- Sea salt and pepper to taste
- 1 tsp garlic powder
- 1 tsp dried rosemary
- 1 tsp Dijon mustard

1. Make a paste in a small bowl by stirring together mustard, garlic powder, rosemary, salt, and pepper.
2. Rub the paste evenly onto the lamb and put it in your slow cooker.
3. Pour in broth, white wine, and onion around the lamb.
4. Cover with the lid and cook for 6 hours on "Low".
5. Serve.

PER SERVING

Cal 780 | Fat 40g | Carbs 3g | Protein 92g

Lamb Meatballs with Dill Sauce

Prep time: 15 minutes | Cook time: 7 to 8 hours | Serves 12

- 1½ pounds ground lamb
- 1 small white onion, minced
- 1 large egg
- 1 teaspoon garlic powder
- ½ teaspoon sea salt
- ½ teaspoon ground cumin
- ½ teaspoon pumpkin pie spice
- ½ teaspoon paprika
- ¼ teaspoon freshly ground black pepper
- 1 cup Avocado-Dill Sauce

1. In a large bowl, combine the lamb, onion, egg, garlic powder, salt, cumin, pumpkin pie spice, paprika, and pepper. Mix well. Form the lamb mixture into about 12 meatballs. Arrange the meatballs along the bottom of your slow cooker.
2. Cover the cooker and set. Cook for 7 to 8 hours.
3. Serve with the avocado-dill sauce.

PER SERVING

Calories: 200 | Total Fat: 17g | Total Carbs: 2g | Sugar: 0g | Fiber: 1g | Protein: 10g | Sodium: 138mg

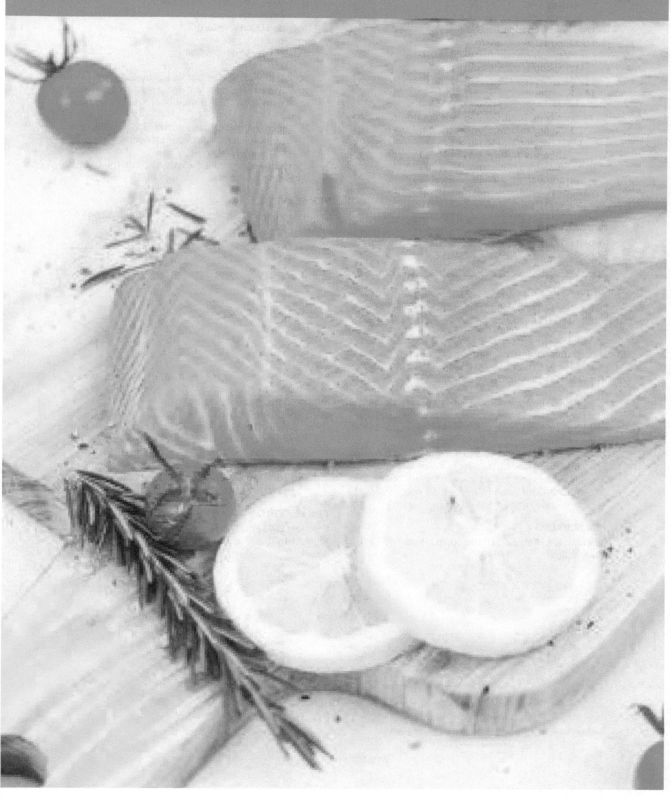

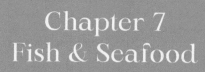
Chapter 7
Fish & Seafood

Keto Wraps with Anchovies

Prep time: 5 minutes | Cook time: 10 minutes | Serves 4

- 2 (2-ounce) can anchovies in olive oil, drained
- 1 cucumber, sliced
- 2 cups red cabbage, shredded
- 1 red onion, chopped
- 1 teaspoon Dijon mustard
- 4 tablespoons mayonnaise
- 1/4 teaspoon ground black pepper
- 1 large-sized tomato, diced
- 12 lettuce leaves

1. In a mixing bowl, combine the anchovies with the cucumber, cabbage, onion, mustard, mayonnaise, black pepper, and tomatoes.
2. Arrange the lettuce leaves on a tray. Spoon the anchovy/vegetable mixture into the center of a lettuce leaf, taco-style.
3. Repeat until you run out of ingredients. Bon appétit!

PER SERVING

Calories: 191 | Fat: 13.3g | Carbs: 6.5g | Protein: 9.9g | Fiber: 2.5g

Grilled Fish Salade Niçoise

Prep time: 5 minutes | Cook time: 15 minutes | Serves 2

- 3/4 pound tuna fillet, skinless
- 1 white onion, sliced
- 1 teaspoon Dijon mustard
- 8 Niçoise olives, pitted and sliced
- 1/2 teaspoon anchovy paste

1. Brush the tuna with nonstick cooking oil; season with salt and freshly cracked black pepper. Then, grill your tuna on a lightly oiled rack approximately 7 minutes, turning over once or twice.
2. Let the fish stand for 3 to 4 minutes and break into bite-sized pieces. Transfer to a nice salad bowl.
3. Toss the tuna pieces with the white onion, Dijon mustard, Niçoise olives, and anchovy paste. Serve well chilled and enjoy!

PER SERVING

Calories: 194 | Fat: 3.4g | Carbs: 0.9g | Protein: 37.1g | Fiber: 0.5g

Grilled Anchovies with Caesar Dressing

Prep time: 5 minutes | Cook time: 15 minutes | Serves 3

- 6 anchovies, cleaned and deboned
- 1 fresh garlic clove, peeled
- 1 teaspoon Dijon mustard
- 2 egg yolks
- 1/3 cup extra-virgin olive oil

1. Place the anchovies onto a lightly oiled grill pan; place under the grill for 2 minutes. Turn them over and cook for a further minute or so; remove from the grill.
2. Process the garlic, Dijon mustard, egg yolks, and extra-virgin olive oil in your blender. Blend until creamy and uniform.
3. Serve the warm grilled anchovies with the Caesar dressing on the side. Bon appétit!

PER SERVING

Calories: 449 | Fat: 34.3g | Carbs: 1g | Protein: 32.6g | Fiber: 0.1g

Fisherman's White Chowder

Prep time: 5 minutes | Cook time: 20 minutes | Serves 4

- 2 teaspoons butter, at room temperature
- 1/2 white onion, chopped
- 1 tablespoon Old Bay seasoning
- 3/4 pound sea bass, broken into chunks
- 1 cup double cream

1. Melt the butter in a soup pot over a moderate flame. Now, sweat the white onion until tender and translucent.
2. Then, add in the Old Bay seasoning and 3 cups of water; bring to a rapid boil. Reduce the heat to medium-low and let it simmer, covered, for 9 to 12 minutes.
3. Fold in the sea bass and double cream; continue to cook until everything is thoroughly heated or about 5 minutes. Serve warm and enjoy!

PER SERVING

Calories: 257 | Fat: 17.8g | Carbs: 3.8g | Protein: 21.3g | Fiber: 0.4g

Mediterranean Salmon

Prep time: 5 minutes | Cook time: 10 minutes | Serves 4

- 4 salmon fillets
- 2 tbsp olive oil
- 1 rosemary sprig
- 1 cup cherry tomatoes
- 15 oz asparagus

1. Pour 1 cup of water into the Instant Pot and insert the steamer rack.
2. Place the salmon on the steamer rack skin side down, rub with rosemary, and arrange the asparagus on top.
3. Seal the lid and cook on "Manual" for 4 minutes.
4. Perform a quick pressure release and carefully open the lid.
5. Add in the cherry tomatoes on top and cook for another 2 minutes.
6. Perform a quick pressure release.
7. Serve drizzled with olive oil.

PER SERVING

Cal 475| Fat 32g| Carbs 6g| Protein 43g

Almond Crusted Tilapia

Prep time: 5 minutes | Cook time: 15 minutes | Serves 4

- 4 tilapia fillets
- 2 tbsp sliced almonds
- 2 tbsp Dijon mustard
- 1 tsp olive oil
- ¼ tsp black pepper

1. Pour 1 cup of water in your Instant Pot.
2. Mix the olive oil, pepper, and mustard in a small bowl.
3. Brush the fish fillets with the mustardy mixture on all sides.
4. Coat the fish in almonds slices.
5. Place the rack in your pot and arrange the fish fillets on it.
6. Close the lid and cook for 5 minutes on "Manual" setting on High pressure.
7. Do a quick pressure release and serve immediately.

PER SERVING

Cal 330| Fat 15g| Carbs 4g| Protein 46g

Ahi Poke With Cucumber

Prep time: 10 minutes | Cook time: 5 minutes | Serves 4

- 1 pound sushi-grade ahi tuna, cut into 1-inch cubes
- 3 scallions, thinly sliced
- 1 serrano chile, seeded and minced (optional)
- 3 tablespoons coconut aminos
- 1 teaspoon rice vinegar
- 1 teaspoon sesame oil
- 1 teaspoon toasted sesame seeds
- Dash ground ginger
- 1 large avocado, diced
- 1 cucumber, sliced into ½-inch-thick rounds

1. In a large bowl, gently mix the tuna, scallions, serrano chile, coconut aminos, vinegar, sesame oil, sesame seeds, and ginger until well combined. Cover and refrigerate to marinate for 15 minutes.
2. Stir in the avocado, gently incorporating the chunks into the ahi mixture.
3. Arrange the cucumber slices on a plate. Place a spoonful of the ahi poke on each cucumber slice and serve immediately.

PER SERVING

Calories: 214 | Total Fat: 15g | Saturated Fat: 2g | Cholesterol: 68mg | Carbohydrates: 11g | Fiber: 4g; | Protein: 10g

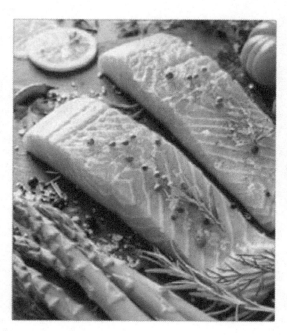

Seared Honey-Garlic Scallops

Prep time: **10 minutes** | Cook time: **15 minutes** | Serves **4**

- 1 pound large scallops, rinsed
- Dash salt
- Dash freshly ground black pepper
- 2 tablespoons avocado oil
- ¼ cup raw honey
- 3 tablespoons coconut aminos
- 2 garlic cloves, minced
- 1 tablespoon apple cider vinegar

1. Pat the scallops dry with paper towels and sprinkle with the salt and pepper.
2. Place the scallops in the skillet, and cook for 2 to 3 minutes per side until golden. Transfer to a plate, tent loosely with aluminum foil to keep warm, and set aside.
3. In the same skillet, stir together the honey, coconut aminos, garlic, and vinegar. Bring to a simmer, and cook for 7 minutes, stirring occasionally as the liquid reduces.
4. Return the scallops to the skillet with the glaze. Toss gently to coat and serve warm.

PER SERVING

Calories: 383 | Total Fat: 19g | Saturated Fat: 3g | Cholesterol: 64mg | Carbohydrates: 26g | Fiber: 1g; | Protein: 21g

Salmon & Asparagus Skewers

Prep time: **15 minutes** | Cook time: **10 minutes** | Serves **8**

- 2 tablespoons ghee, melted
- 1 teaspoon Dijon mustard
- 1 teaspoon garlic powder
- ½ teaspoon salt
- ¼ teaspoon red pepper flakes
- 1½ pounds boned skinless salmon, cut into 2-inch chunks
- 2 lemons, thinly sliced
- 1 bunch asparagus spears, tough ends trimmed, cut into 2-inch pieces

1. Preheat the broiler.
2. Line a baking sheet with aluminum foil.
3. In a small saucepan over medium heat, heat the ghee.
4. On each skewer, thread 1 chunk of salmon, 1 lemon slice folded in half, and 2 pieces of asparagus. Repeat with the remaining skewers until all ingredients are used. Place the skewers on the prepared pan and brush each with the ghee-seasoning mixture.
5. Broil for 4 minutes. Turn the skewers and broil on the other side for about 4 minutes.

PER SERVING

Calories: 250 | Total Fat: 9g | Saturated Fat: 5g | Cholesterol: 68mg | Carbohydrates: 4g | Fiber: 2g; | Protein: 38g

Hawaiian Tuna

Prep time: **5 minutes** | Cook time: **30 minutes** | Serves **4**

- 2 lb tuna, cubed
- 1 cup pineapple chunks
- ¼ cup chopped cilantro
- 2 tbsp chopped parsley
- 2 garlic cloves, minced
- 1 tbsp coconut oil
- 1 tbsp coconut aminos
- Sea salt and pepper to taste

1. Preheat your oven to 400°F.
2. Add the tuna, pineapple, cilantro, parsley, garlic, coconut aminos, salt, and pepper to a baking dish and stir to coat.
3. Bake for 15-20 minutes, or until the fish feels firm to the touch.
4. Serve warm.

PER SERVING

Cal 410| Fat 15g| Carbs 7g| Protein 59g

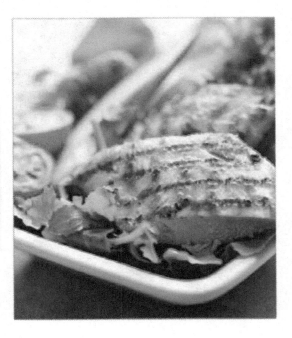

Avocado & Tuna Toast

Prep time: 5 minutes | Cook time: 10 minutes | Serves 4

- 2 (5-oz) cans wild-caught albacore tuna
- 1 shallot, minced
- 4 sourdough bread slices
- ¼ cup paleo mayonnaise
- 1 tsp lemon juice
- ¼ tsp paprika
- 1 avocado, cut into 8 slices
- 1 tomato, cut into 8 slices
- 3 tsp grated Parmesan cheese

1. Preheat your broiler to high.
2. Line a baking sheet with foil.
3. Place the bread slices on the sheet.
4. Combine the mayonnaise, tuna, lemon juice, shallot, and paprika in a bowl and put it on top of each slice.
5. Add in 2 tomato slices and 2 avocado slices on each bread and scatter with 1 tbsp of Parmesan cheese.
6. Place the sheet in the broil and cook for 3-4 minutes.
7. Serve immediately.

PER SERVING

Cal 470| Fat 28g| Carbs 30g| Protein 27g

Cod in Tomato Sauce

Prep time: 5 minutes | Cook time: 10 minutes | Serves 4

- 4 cod fillets
- 2 cups chopped tomatoes
- 1 tbsp olive oil
- Sea salt and pepper to taste
- ¼ tsp garlic powder

1. Place the tomatoes in a baking dish and crush them with a fork.
2. Season with some salt, pepper, and garlic powder.
3. Season the cod with salt and pepper and place it over the tomatoes.
4. Drizzle the olive oil over the fish and tomatoes.
5. Add 1 cup of water and a trivet in your Instant Pot.
6. Place the baking dish on the trivet.
7. Close the lid and cook on "Manual" for 10 minutes.
8. Once the timer goes off, let the steam release naturally for about 10 minutes before releasing the remaining pressure manually.
9. Serve.

PER SERVING

Cal 250| Fat 5g| Carbs 3g| Protein 45g

Goan Curried Fish Stew

Prep time: 5 minutes | Cook time: 25 minutes |Serves 3

- 1 tablespoon butter, at room temperature
- 1 shallot, chopped
- 1 teaspoon curry paste
- 1 cup tomatoes, pureed
- 3/4 pound sole fillets, cut into 1-inch pieces

1. Melt the butter in a stockpot over a medium-high flame. Sauté the shallot until softened.
2. Add the curry paste and pureed tomatoes along with 2 cups of water to the pot; bring to a rolling boil.
3. Immediately reduce the heat to medium-low and continue to simmer, covered, for 12 minutes longer; make sure to stir periodically.
4. Fold in the chopped sole fillets; continue to cook for a further 8 minutes or until the fish flakes easily with a fork. Enjoy!

PER SERVING

Calories: 191 | Fat: 9.1g | Carbs: 2.8g | Protein: 23.9g | Fiber: 1.1g

Spanish Fish à La Nage

Prep time: 5 minutes | Cook time: 20 minutes |Serves 5

- 2 tablespoons olive oil
- 1 Spanish onion, chopped
- 1 medium-sized zucchini, diced
- 2 vine-ripe tomatoes, pureed
- 1 ½ pounds cod fish fillets

1. Heat the olive oil in a stockpot over medium-high flame. Now, cook the Spanish onion until tender and translucent.
2. Pour in the pureed tomatoes along with 2 cups of water. Bring to a boil and reduce the heat to medium-low. Let it simmer an additional 10 to 13 minutes.
3. Now, fold in the cod fish fillets. Cook, covered, an additional 5 to 6 minutes or until the codfish is just cooked through and an instant-read thermometer registers 140 degrees F.
4. Place the fish in individual bowls; ladle the fish broth over each serving, and serve hot.
5. Enjoy!

PER SERVING

Calories: 177 | Fat: 6.4g | Carbs: 4g | Protein: 24.9g | Fiber: 1g

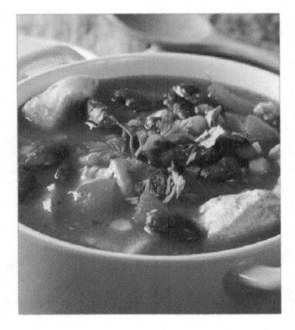

Coconut-Crusted Shrimp

Prep time: 10 minutes | Cook time: 6 minutes | Serves 4

- 2 eggs
- 1 cup unsweetened dried coconut
- ¼ cup coconut flour
- ½ teaspoon salt
- ¼ teaspoon paprika
- Dash cayenne pepper
- Dash freshly ground black pepper
- ¼ cup coconut oil
- 1 pound raw shrimp, peeled and deveined

1. In a small shallow bowl, whisk the eggs.
2. In another small shallow bowl, mix the coconut, coconut flour, salt, paprika, cayenne pepper, and black pepper.
3. In a large skillet over medium-high heat, heat the coconut oil.
4. Pat the shrimp dry with a paper towel.
5. Working one at a time, hold each shrimp by the tail, dip it into the egg mixture, and then into the coconut mixture until coated. Place into the hot skillet. Cook for 1 to 3 minutes per side. Transfer to a paper towel–lined plate to drain excess oil.
6. Serve immediately.

PER SERVING

Calories: 279 | Total Fat: 2 0g | Saturated Fat: 15g | Cholesterol: 258mg | Carbohydrates: 6g | Fiber: 3g; | Protein: 19g

Summer Salad with Cod Fish

Prep time: 5 minutes | Cook time:15 minutes |Serves 5

- 4 tablespoons extra-virgin olive oil
- 5 cod fillets
- 1/4 cup balsamic vinegar
- 1 tablespoon stone-ground mustard
- Sea salt and ground black pepper, to season
- 1/2 pound green cabbage, shredded
- 2 cups lettuce, cut into small pieces
- 1 red onion, sliced
- 1 garlic clove, minced
- 1 teaspoon red pepper flakes

1. Heat 1 tablespoon of the olive oil in a large frying pan over medium-high heat.
2. Once hot, fry the fish fillets for 5 minutes until golden brown; flip them and cook on the other side for 4 to 5 minutes more; work in batches to avoid overcrowding the pan.
3. Flake the cod fillets with two forks and reserve.
4. To make the dressing, whisk the remaining tablespoon of olive oil with the balsamic vinegar, mustard, salt, and black pepper.
5. Combine the green cabbage, lettuce, onion, and garlic in a salad bowl. Dress the salad and top with the reserved fish.
6. Garnish with red pepper flakes and serve. Enjoy!

PER SERVING

Calories: 276 | Fat: 6.9g | Carbs: 6.4g | Protein: 42.7g | Fiber: 1.7g

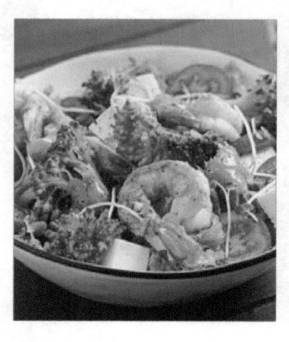

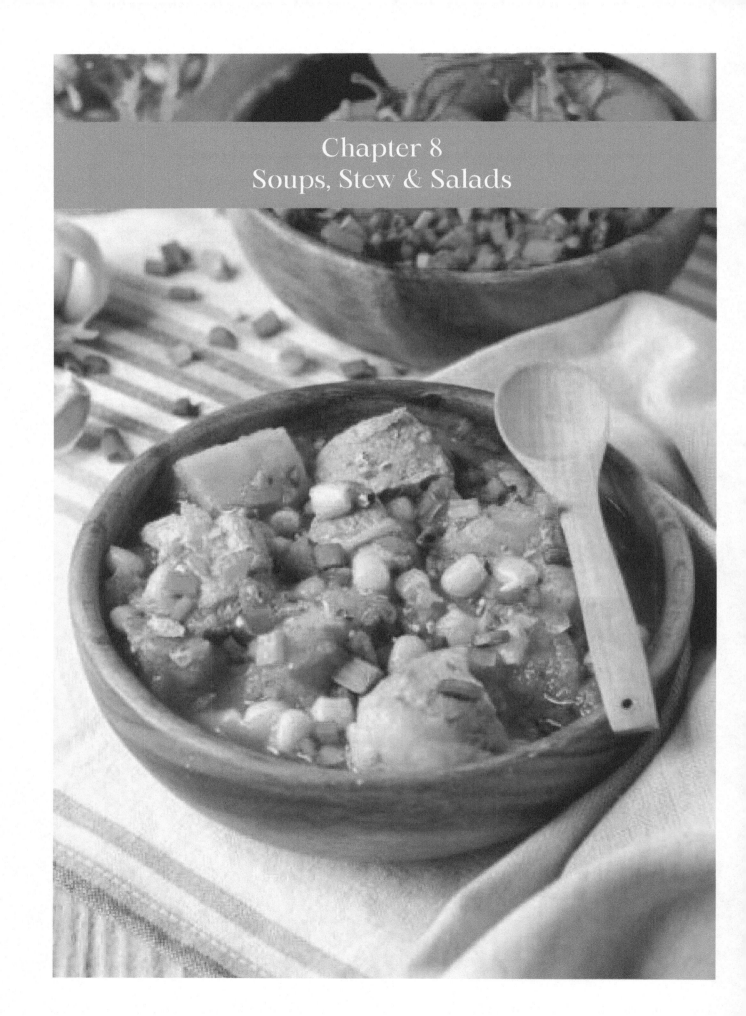

Chapter 8
Soups, Stew & Salads

Homemade Cold Gazpacho Soup

Prep time: 15 minutes | Cook time: 5 minutes | Serves 6

- 2 small green peppers, roasted
- 2 large red peppers, roasted
- 2 medium avocados, flesh scoped out
- 2 garlic cloves
- 2 spring onions, chopped
- 1 cucumber, chopped
- cup olive oil
- tbsp lemon juice
- 4 tomatoes, chopped
- 7 ounces goat cheese
- small red onion, chopped
- tbsp apple cider vinegar
- Salt to taste

1. Place the peppers, tomatoes, avocados, red onion, garlic, lemon juice, olive oil, vinegar, and salt, in a food processor. Pulse until your desired consistency is reached. Taste and adjust the seasoning.
2. Transfer the mixture to a pot. Stir in cucumber and spring onions. Cover and chill in the fridge at least 2 hours. Divide the soup between 6 bowls. Serve topped with goat cheese and an extra drizzle of olive oil.

PER SERVING

Kcal: 528 | Fat: 45.8g | Net Carbs: 6.5g | Protein: 7.5g

Cream of Thyme Tomato Soup

Prep time: 20 minutes | Cook time: 14 minutes | Serves 6

- 2 tbsp ghee
- 2 large red onions, diced
- ½ cup raw cashew nuts, diced
- 2 (28 oz) cans tomatoes
- 1 tsp fresh thyme leaves + extra to garnish
- 1½ cups water
- Salt and black pepper to taste
- 1 cup heavy cream

1. Melt ghee in a pot over medium heat and sauté the onions for 4 minutes until softened.
2. Stir in the tomatoes, thyme, water, cashews, and season with salt and black pepper. Cover and bring to simmer for 10 minutes until thoroughly cooked.
3. Open, turn the heat off, and puree the ingredients with an immersion blender. Adjust to taste and stir in the heavy cream. Spoon into soup bowls and serve.

PER SERVING

Kcal: 310 | Fat: 27g | Net Carbs: 3g | Protein: 11g

Green Minestrone Soup

Prep time: 25 minutes | Cook time: 11 minutes | Serves 4

- tbsp ghee
- 2 tbsp onion-garlic puree
- 2 heads broccoli, cut in florets
- 2 stalks celery, chopped
- 5 cups vegetable broth
- cup baby spinach
- Salt and black pepper to taste
- tbsp Gruyere cheese, grated

1. Melt the ghee in a saucepan over medium heat and sauté the onion-garlic puree for 3 minutes until softened. Mix in the broccoli and celery, and cook for 4 minutes until slightly tender. Pour in the broth, bring to a boil, then reduce the heat to medium-low and simmer covered for about 5 minutes.
2. Drop in the spinach to wilt, adjust the seasonings, and cook for 4 minutes. Ladle soup into serving bowls. Serve with a sprinkle of grated Gruyere cheese.

PER SERVING

Kcal: 227 | Fat: 20.3g | Net Carbs: 2g | Protein: 8g

Creamy Cauliflower Soup with Bacon Chips

Prep time: 25 minutes | Cook time: 13 minutes | Serves 4

- 2 tbsp ghee
- onion, chopped
- head cauliflower, cut into florets
- cups water
- Salt and black pepper to taste
- cups almond milk
- 1 cup shredded white cheddar cheese
- 3 bacon strips

1. Melt the ghee in a saucepan over medium heat and sauté the onion for 3 minutes until fragrant.
2. Include the cauli florets, sauté for 3 minutes to slightly soften, add the water, and season with salt and black pepper. Bring to a boil, and then reduce the heat to low. Cover and cook for 10 minutes. Puree cauliflower with an immersion blender until the ingredients are evenly combined and stir in the almond milk and cheese until the cheese melts. Adjust taste with salt and black pepper.
3. In a non-stick skillet over high heat, fry the bacon, until crispy. Divide soup between serving bowls, top with crispy bacon, and serve hot.

PER SERVING

Kcal: 402 | Fat: 37g | Net Carbs: 6g | Protein: 8g

Chickpea and Kale Salad
Prep time: 10 minutes | Cooking time: 20 minutes | Serves 4

- 1 large bunch kale, thoroughly washed, stemmed, and cut into thin strips
- 2 teaspoons freshly squeezed lemon juice
- 2 tablespoons extra-virgin olive oil, divided
- ¾ teaspoon sea salt, divided
- 2 cups cooked chickpeas (about 1 [14-oz] can)
- 1 teaspoon sweet paprika
- 1 avocado, chopped (optional)

1. In a large bowl, combine the kale, lemon juice, 1 tablespoon of olive oil, and ¼ teaspoon of salt.
2. With your hands, massage the kale for 5 minutes, or until it starts to wilt and becomes bright green and shiny.
3. To a skillet set over medium-low heat, add the remaining 1 tablespoon of olive oil.
4. Stir in the chickpeas, paprika, and remaining ½ teaspoon of salt. Cook for about 15 minutes, or until warm. The chickpeas might start to crisp in spots.
5. Pour the chickpeas over the kale. Toss well. Add the avocado (if using).
6. Serve immediately.

PER SERVING:

Calories: 359| Total Fat: 20g| Total Carbohydrates: 35g| Sugar: 1g| Fiber: 10g| Protein: 13g| Sodium: 497mg

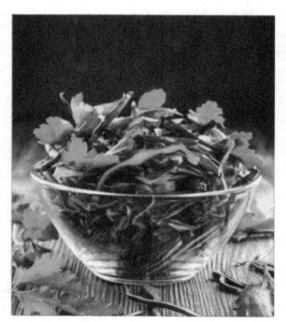

Thyme & Wild Mushroom Soup
Prep time: 25 minutes | Cook time: 20 minutes | Serves 4

- ¼ cup butter
- ½ cup crème fraiche
- 12 oz wild mushrooms, chopped
- 2 tsp thyme leaves
- 2 garlic cloves, minced
- 4 cups chicken broth
- Salt and black pepper, to taste

1. Melt the butter in a large pot over medium heat. Add garlic and cook for one minute until tender. Add mushrooms, salt and pepper, and cook for 10 minutes. Pour the broth over and bring to a boil.
2. Reduce the heat and simmer for 10 minutes. Puree the soup with a hand blender until smooth. Stir in crème fraiche. Garnish with thyme leaves before serving.

PER SERVING

Kcal: 281 | Fat: 25g | Net Carbs: 5.8g | Protein: 6.1g

Chicken Creamy Soup
Prep time: 15 minutes | Cook time: 5 minutes | Serves 4

- 2 cups cooked and shredded chicken
- 3 tbsp butter, melted
- 4 cups chicken broth
- 4 tbsp chopped cilantro ⅓ cup buffalo sauce
- ½ cup cream cheese
- Salt and black pepper, to taste

1. Blend the butter, buffalo sauce, and cream cheese, in a food processor, until smooth. Transfer to a pot, add chicken broth and heat until hot but do not bring to a boil.
2. Stir in chicken, salt, black pepper and cook until heated through. When ready, remove to soup bowls and serve garnished with cilantro.

PER SERVING

Kcal: 406 | Fat: 29.5g | Net Carbs: 5g | Protein: 26.5g

Cobb Egg Salad in Lettuce Cups

Prep time: 25 minutes | **Cook time:** 18 minutes | **Serves 4**

- 2 chicken breasts, cut into pieces
- 1 tbsp olive oil
- Salt and black pepper to season
- 6 large eggs
- 1½ cups water
- 2 tomatoes, seeded, chopped
- 6 tbsp Greek yogurt
- 1 head green lettuce, firm leaves removed for cups

1. Preheat oven to 400°F. Put the chicken pieces in a bowl, drizzle with olive oil, and sprinkle with salt and black pepper. Mix the ingredients until the chicken is well coated with the seasoning.
2. Put the chicken on a prepared baking sheet and spread out evenly. Slide the baking sheet in the oven and bake the chicken until cooked through and golden brown for 8 minutes, turning once.
3. Bring the eggs to boil in salted water in a pot over medium heat for 10 minutes. Run the eggs in cold water, peel, and chop into small pieces. Transfer to a salad bowl.
4. Remove the chicken from the oven when ready and add to the salad bowl. Include the tomatoes and Greek yogurt; mix evenly with a spoon. Layer two lettuce leaves each as cups and fill with two tablespoons of egg salad each. Serve with chilled blueberry juice.

PER SERVING

Kcal: 325 | Fat: 24.5g | Net Carbs: 4g | Protein: 21g

Thai Sweet Potato Soup

Prep time: 10 minutes | **Cooking time:** 20 minutes | **Serves 4 to 6**

- 3 large sweet potatoes, cubed
- 2 cups water
- 1 (14-ounce) can coconut milk
- ½-inch piece fresh ginger, sliced
- ½ cup almond butter
- Zest of 1 lime
- Juice of 1 lime
- 1 teaspoon salt, plus additional as needed

1. In a large pot set over high heat, combine the sweet potatoes, water, coconut milk, and ginger. Bring to a boil. Reduce the heat to low and cover.
2. Simmer for 20 to 25 minutes, or until the potatoes are tender. Transfer the potatoes, ginger, and cooking liquid to a blender.
3. Add the almond butter, lime zest, lime juice, and salt.
4. Blend until smooth.
5. Taste, and adjust the seasoning if necessary.

PER SERVING:

Calories: 653| Total Fat: 42g| Total Carbohydrates: 64g| Sugar: 4g| Fiber: 11g| Protein: 12g| Sodium: 614mg

Tuna Caprese Salad

Prep time: 10 minutes | **Cook time:** 5 minutes | **Serves 4**

- 2 (10 oz) cans tuna chunks in water, drained
- 2 tomatoes, sliced
- 8 oz fresh mozzarella cheese, sliced
- 6 basil leaves
- ½ cup black olives, pitted and sliced
- 2 tbsp extra virgin olive oil
- ½ lemon, juiced

1. Place the tuna in the center of a serving platter. Arrange the cheese and tomato slices around the tuna. Alternate a slice of tomato, cheese, and a basil leaf.
2. To finish, scatter the black olives over the top, drizzle with olive oil and lemon juice and serve.

PER SERVING

Kcal: 360 | Fat: 31g | Net Carbs: 1g | Protein: 21g

Classic Butternut Squash Soup

Prep time: 20 minutes | **Cooking time:** 30 minutes | **Serves 6**

- 1 onion, roughly chopped
- 4½ cups plus 2 tablespoons water, divided
- 1 large butternut squash, washed, peeled, ends trimmed, halved, seeded, and cut into ½-inch chunks
- 2 celery stalks, roughly chopped
- 3 carrots, peeled and roughly chopped
- 1 teaspoon sea salt, plus additional as needed

1. In a large pot set over medium heat, sauté the onion in 2 tablespoons of water for about 5 minutes, or until soft.
2. Add the squash, celery, carrot, and salt. Bring to a boil.
3. Reduce the heat to low, Cover and simmer for 25 minutes.
4. In a blender, purée the soup until smooth, working in batches if necessary and taking care with the hot liquid. Taste, and adjust the seasoning if necessary.

PER SERVING:

Calories: 104| Total Fat: 0g| Total Carbohydrates: 27g| Sugar: 6g| Fiber: 5g| Protein: 2g| Sodium: 417mg

Mediterranean Salad
Prep time: 10 minutes | Cook time: 5 minutes | Serves 4

- 3 tomatoes, sliced
- 1 large avocado, sliced
- 8 kalamata olives
- ¼ lb buffalo mozzarella cheese, sliced
- 2 tbsp pesto sauce 2 tbsp olive oil

1. Arrange the tomato slices on a serving platter and place the avocado slices in the middle.
2. Arrange the olives around the avocado slices and drop pieces of mozzarella on the platter.
3. Drizzle the pesto sauce all over, and drizzle olive oil as well.

PER SERVING
Kcal: 290 | Fat: 25g | Net Carbs: 4.3g | Protein: 9g

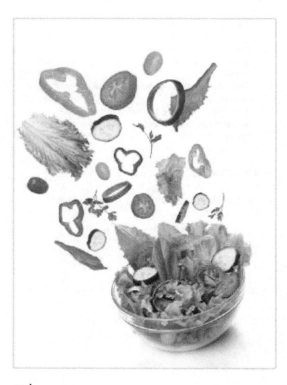

Glorious Creamed Greens Soup
Prep time: 10 minutes | Cooking time: 15 minutes | Serves 4 to 6

- 3 cups water
- 2 cups unsweetened coconut milk
- 4 cups tightly packed kale, thoroughly washed, stemmed, and roughly chopped
- 4 cups tightly packed spinach, stemmed and roughly chopped
- 4 cups tightly packed collard greens, stemmed and roughly chopped
- 1 bunch fresh parsley, stemmed and roughly chopped

1. In a large pot set over high heat, bring the water, coconut milk, and salt to a boil. Reduce the heat to low.
2. Add the kale, spinach, and collard greens 1 cup at a time, letting them wilt before adding the next cup. Continue until all the greens have been added to the pot.
3. Simmer for 8 to 10 minutes.
4. Taste, and adjust the seasoning (if necessary) before serving.

PER SERVING:
Calories: 334| Total Fat: 29g| Total Carbohydrates: 18g| Sugar: 4g| Fiber: 6g| Protein: 7g| Sodium: 959mg

Lentil Bolognese
Prep time: 15 minutes | Cook time: 30 minutes | Serves 4 to 6

- 1 tablespoon extra-virgin olive oil
- 2 carrots, grated
- 1 celery stalk, minced
- 1 small onion, diced
- ½ teaspoon garlic powder
- 4 cups diced tomatoes
- 1 cup lentils, soaked in water overnight, drained, and rinsed well
- 1 bay leaf
- ½ teaspoon dried oregano
- ½ teaspoon dried basil leaves
- ½ teaspoon sea salt
- ¼ teaspoon red pepper flakes
- ¼ teaspoon ground nutmeg
- Freshly ground black pepper

1. Coat the slow cooker with the olive oil. Add the carrots, celery, onion, and garlic powder.
2. Cover the cooker and set to high. Cook for 30 minutes.
3. Stir in the tomatoes, broth, lentils, bay leaf, oregano, basil, salt, red pepper flakes, and nutmeg, then season with black pepper. Re-cover the cooker and set to low. Cook for 5 to 6 hours.
4. Remove and discard the bay leaf before serving.

PER SERVING
Calories: 180 | Total Fat: 4g | Total Carbs: 35g | Sugar: 5g | Fiber: 15g | Protein: 12g | Sodium: 607mg

Radish & Cabbage Ginger Salad

Prep time: 5 minutes | Cook time: 10 minutes | Serves 4

- 8 oz napa cabbage, cut crosswise into strips
- 2 tbsp chopped roasted hazelnuts
- 1 cup grated carrots
- 1 cup sliced radishes
- 2 green onions, minced
- 2 tbsp chopped parsley
- 2 tbsp rice vinegar
- 2 tsp olive oil
- 1 tsp low-sodium soy sauce
- 1 tsp grated fresh ginger
- ½ tsp dry mustard
- Sea salt and pepper to taste

1. Place the cabbage, carrot, radishes, green onions, and parsley in a bowl, stir to combine.
2. In another bowl, mix vinegar, olive oil, soy sauce, ginger, mustard, salt, and pepper.
3. Pour over the slaw and toss to coat.
4. Place in the fridge for 2 hours.
5. Serve topped with hazelnuts.

PER SERVING

Cal 80| Fat 6g| Carbs 6g| Protein 10g

Easy Pineapple & Jicama Salad

Prep time: 5 minutes | Cook time: 10 minutes | Serves 6

- 1 jicama, peeled and grated
- 1 peeled pineapple, sliced
- ¼ cup non-dairy milk
- 2 tbsp fresh basil, chopped
- 1 large scallion, chopped
- Sea salt to taste
- 1½ tbsp tahini
- Arugula for serving
- Chopped cashews

1. Place jicama in a bowl.
2. In a food processor, put the pineapple and enough milk.
3. Blitz until puréed.
4. Add in basil, scallions, tahini, and salt.
5. Pour over the jicama and cover.
6. Transfer to the fridge and marinate for 1 hour.
7. Place a bed of arugula on a plate and top with the salad.
8. Serve garnished with cashews.

PER SERVING

Cal 175| Fat 5g| Carbs 33g| Protein 2g

Broccoli & Mango Rice Salad

Prep time: 5 minutes | Cook time: 20 minutes | Serves 4

- 3 cups broccoli florets, blanched
- 1/3 cup roasted almonds, chopped
- ½ cup brown rice, rinsed
- 1 mango, chopped
- 1 red bell pepper, chopped
- 1 jalapeño, minced
- 1 tsp grated fresh ginger
- 2 tbsp fresh lemon juice
- 3 tbsp grapeseed oil

1. Place the rice in a bowl with salted water and cook for 18-20 minutes.
2. Remove to a bowl.
3. Stir in broccoli, mango, bell pepper, and chili.
4. In another bowl, mix the ginger, lemon juice, and oil.
5. Pour over the rice and toss to combine.
6. Top with almonds.
7. Serve and enjoy!

PER SERVING

Cal 290| Fat 15g| Carbs 35g| Protein 1g

Kale & White Bean Chili

Prep time: 15 minutes | Cook time: 6 to 8 hours | Serves 4 to 6

- 2 cups dried cannellini beans, soaked in water overnight, drained, and rinsed well
- 1 small bunch kale, washed, chopped, and de-ribbed
- 1 small onion, diced
- ½ green bell pepper, seeded and chopped
- 1 (4-ounce) can Hatch green chiles
- 4 cups vegetable broth
- ½ teaspoon garlic powder
- 1 teaspoon chili powder
- ½ teaspoon ground cumin
- 2 tablespoons extra-virgin olive oil
- 1 avocado, peeled, pitted, and chopped

1. In your slow cooker, combine the beans, kale, onion, bell pepper, chiles, broth, garlic powder, chili powder, and cumin. Stir to mix the ingredients.
2. Cover the cooker and set to low. Cook for 6 to 8 hours.
3. Drizzle each bowl with olive oil, top with avocado, and serve.

PER SERVING

Calories: 476 | Total Fat: 16g | Total Carbs: 67g | Sugar: 3g | Fiber: 13g | Protein: 22g | Sodium: 589mg

Classic Vegetable Broth

Prep time: 15 minutes | Cook time: 6 to 8 hours | Serves 12

- Extra-virgin olive oil, for coating the slow cooker
- 6 cups veggie scraps (peels and pieces of carrots, celery, onions, garlic)
- 12 cups filtered water
- ½ medium onion, roughly chopped
- 2 garlic cloves, roughly chopped
- 1 parsley sprig
- ¾ teaspoon sea salt
- ½ teaspoon dried oregano
- ½ teaspoon dried basil leaves
- 2 bay leaves

1. Coat the slow cooker with a thin layer of olive oil.
2. In the slow cooker, combine the veggie scraps, water, onion, garlic, parsley, salt, oregano, basil, and bay leaves.
3. Cover the cooker and set to low. Cook for 6 to 8 hours.
4. Pour the broth through a fine-mesh sieve set over a large bowl, discarding the veggie scraps. Refrigerate the broth in airtight containers for up to 5 days, or freeze for up to 3 months.

PER SERVING

Calories: 24 | Total Fat: 0g | Total Carbs: 5g | Sugar: 2g | Fiber: 1g | Protein: 1g | Sodium: 202mg

Masala Lentils

Prep time: 15 minutes | Cook time: 4 to 5 hours | Serves 4 to 6

- 1 cup red lentils, soaked in water overnight, drained, and rinsed well
- 1 (15-ounce) can diced tomatoes
- 1 medium onion, diced
- 2 cups vegetable broth
- 2 teaspoons garam masala
- 1 teaspoon garlic powder
- 1 teaspoon ground ginger
- 1 teaspoon molasses
- 1 teaspoon sea salt
- ½ teaspoon paprika
- ½ teaspoon ground turmeric
- Pinch cayenne pepper
- Freshly ground black pepper
- 1 cup fresh spinach, roughly chopped
- 1 cup full-fat coconut milk

1. In your slow cooker, combine the lentils, tomatoes, onion, broth, garam masala, garlic powder, ginger, molasses, salt, paprika, turmeric, and cayenne, and season with black pepper.
2. Cover the cooker and set to low. Cook for 4 to 5 hours.
3. Stir in the spinach and re-cover the cooker for 5 minutes to let the spinach wilt.
4. Add the coconut milk, stir, and serve.

PER SERVING

Calories: 232 | Total Fat: 11g | Total Carbs: 32g | Sugar: 8g | Fiber: 13g | Protein: 12g | Sodium: 1,095mg

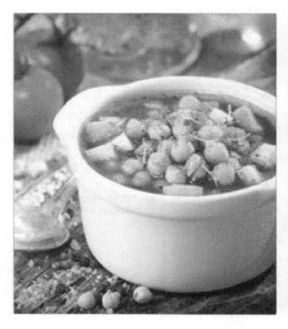
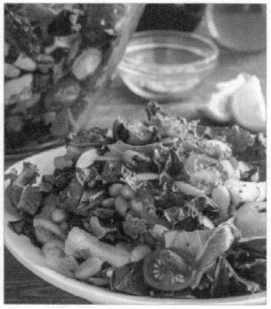

Chapter 9
Dessert

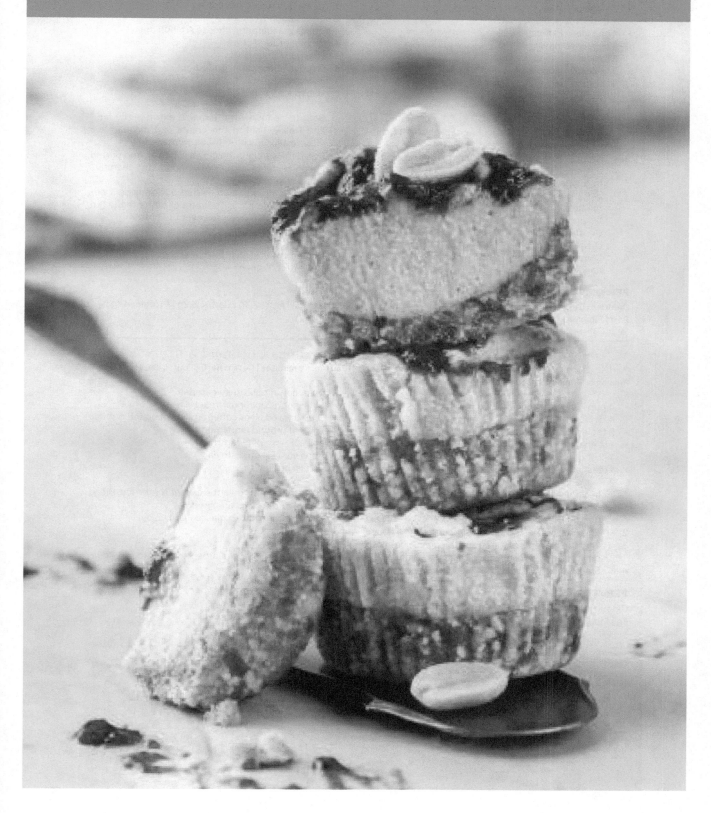

Blueberry Peach Cobbler

Prep time: 15 minutes | Cook time: 2 hours | SERVES 4 TO 6

- 5 tablespoons coconut oil, divided
- 3 large peaches, peeled and sliced
- 2 cups frozen blueberries
- 1 cup almond flour
- 1 cup rolled oats
- 1 tablespoon maple syrup
- 1 tablespoon coconut sugar
- 1 teaspoon ground cinnamon
- ½ teaspoon vanilla extract
- Pinch ground nutmeg

1. Coat the bottom of your slow cooker with 1 tablespoon of coconut oil.
2. Arrange the peaches and blueberries along the bottom of the slow cooker.
3. In a small bowl, stir together the almond flour, oats, remaining 4 tablespoons of coconut oil, maple syrup, coconut sugar, cinnamon, vanilla, and nutmeg until a coarse mixture forms. Gently crumble the topping over the fruit in the slow cooker.
4. Cover the cooker and set to high. Cook for 2 hours and serve.

PER SERVING

Calories: 516 | Total Fat: 34g | Total Carbs: 49g | Sugar: 24g | Fiber: 10g | Protein: 10g | Sodium: 1mg

Warm Cinnamon Turmeric Almond Milk

Prep time: 15 minutes | Cook time: 3 to 4 hours | Serves 4 to 6

- 4 cups unsweetened almond milk
- 4 cinnamon sticks
- 2 tablespoons coconut oil
- 1 (4-inch) piece turmeric root, roughly chopped
- 1 (2-inch) piece fresh ginger, roughly chopped
- 1 teaspoon raw honey, plus more to taste

1. In your slow cooker, combine the almond milk, cinnamon sticks, coconut oil, turmeric, and ginger.
2. Cover the cooker and set to low. Cook for 3 to 4 hours.
3. Pour the contents of the cooker through a fine-mesh sieve into a clean container; discard the solids.
4. Starting with just 1 teaspoon, add raw honey to taste.

PER SERVING

Calories: 133 | Total Fat: 11g | Total Carbs: 10g | Sugar: 7g | Fiber: 1g | Protein: 1g | Sodium: 152mg

Traditional Spanish Frisuelos

Prep time: 5 minutes | Cook time: 20 minutes | Serves 6

- 3 eggs
- 1/2 teaspoon maple extract
- 2 ounces double cream
- 4 ounces mascarpone cheese A pinch of salt
- A pinch of ground cloves
- 1 tablespoon cognac
- 1 teaspoon lemon zest, grated
- 1 tablespoon butter, melted
- 6 tablespoons confectioners' Swerve

1. Beat the eggs with the maple extract until light and frothy. Fold in the cream and mascarpone cheese. Mix again until well combined.
2. Stir in the salt, ground cloves, cognac, and grated lemon zest. Mix again until smooth and there aren't any lumps.
3. Coat a frying pan with melted butter using a paper towel. Add a small amount of batter to the hot pan and spread it out to cover the bottom.
4. Cook for about 2 minutes on each side. Transfer your frisuelo to a large plate and sprinkle confectioners' Swerve on top. Repeat until you run out of the batter. Enjoy!

PER SERVING

Calories: 137 | Fat: 12.3g | Carbs: 3.2g | Protein: 4.1g | Fiber: 0g

Iced Vanilla Coconut Latte

Prep time: 5 minutes | Cook time: 5 minutes | Serves 2

- 1 cup coconut milk, unsweetened
- 4 tablespoons coconut cream
- 1/2 cup brewed black coffee A pinch of grated nutmeg
- A pinch of ground cinnamon
- 1 vanilla bean, split lengthwise
- 8 drops vanilla liquid stevia
- 1 cup ice, crushed

1. Blend all the ingredients, except for the ice. Blend on high until well combined.
2. Divide between two glasses and enjoy!

PER SERVING

Calories: 345 | Fat: 35.3g | Carbs: 6.3g | Protein: 3.4g | Fiber: 3.3g

Classic Chocolate Sheet Cake

Prep time: 10 minutes | Cook time:30 minutes |Serves 8

- 1/2 cup coconut flour 1/2 cup almond meal
- 1/2 teaspoon baking powder
- 1/4 teaspoon ground cinnamon
- 1/4 cup cocoa powder, unsweetened
- 3 eggs
- 1/3 cup coconut oil
- 1/4 cup powdered erythritol 1/2 teaspoon butterscotch extract Ganache:
- 1 avocado, mashed
- 2 tablespoons cocoa powder, unsweetened
- 2 tablespoons coconut oil
- 4 tablespoons coconut milk, unsweetened
- 1/2 teaspoon vanilla paste
- 4 tablespoons powdered erythritol

1. Mix the coconut flour, almond meal, baking powder, ground cinnamon, and cocoa powder until well combined. Gradually, add in the eggs, coconut oil, powdered erythritol, and butterscotch extract.
2. Scrape the batter into a parchment-lined baking pan. Bake in the preheated oven at 320 degrees F for 19 to 22 minutes or until a tester comes out dry and clean.
3. Let your cake cool completely at room temperature.
4. In the meantime, make your ganache by mixing all the ingredients in your blender or food processor. Frost the cake and serve chilled. Enjoy!

PER SERVING

Calories: 244 | Fat: 23.4g | Carbs: 7g | Protein: 5.4g | Fiber: 5.1g

Seedy Cookie Dough Bites

Prep time: 12 minutes | Cooking time: 0 minutes | Serves 4 to 6

- ⅔ cup pumpkin seeds
- ⅔ cup sunflower seeds
- ⅔ cup gluten-free rolled oats
- ¼ cup maple syrup
- 1 teaspoon vanilla extract
- ¼ cup cacao nibs, or dairy-free chocolate chips

1. Line a large plate with parchment paper.
2. In a food processor, combine the pumpkin seeds, sunflower seeds, and oats. Process into a fine meal.
3. Add the maple syrup and vanilla. Blend until combined.
4. Add the cacao nibs and pulse together.
5. Using a 1-tablespoon measure, roll 12-16 cookie balls with your hands. Place them on the prepared plate.
6. Freeze the dough balls for 30 minutes to firm. Transfer to a sealed container. Refrigerate.

PER SERVING:

Calories: 345| Total Fat: 19g| Total Carbohydrates: 36g| Sugar: 12g| Fiber: 6g| Protein: 12g| Sodium: 7mg

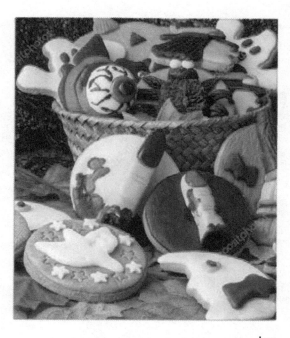

Strawberry Jam Thumbprint Cookies

Prep time: 15 minutes | **Cooking time:** 15 minutes | **Serves 4 to 6**

- 1½ cups sunflower seeds
- 3 tablespoons coconut oil
- ¼ cup maple syrup
- ½ cup strawberry jam, divided

1. Preheat the oven to 350°F.
2. Line a baking sheet with parchment paper.
3. In a blender, food processor, or spice grinder, process the sunflower seeds into a fine meal. Transfer to a large bowl.
4. Add the coconut oil, mashing it into the sunflower meal with a spoon as if you are crumbling butter into flour. Stir in the maple syrup. Mix well.
5. Using a tablespoon measure, scoop the dough onto the prepared sheet, making 12 cookies. Gently press down on the cookies with the back of a wet spoon to flatten them.
6. With your thumb, make imprints in the center of each cookie. Fill each depression with 2 teaspoons of strawberry jam.
7. Place the sheet in the preheated oven and bake for 12 to 14 minutes.
8. Cool before eating.

PER SERVING:

Calories: 392| Total Fat: 19g| Total Carbohydrates: 54g| Sugar: 12g| Fiber: 2g| Protein: 4g| Sodium: 3mg

Coconut Blueberry Popsicles

Prep time: 15 minutes | **Cooking time:** 0 minutes | **Serves 6**

- 1 cup fresh blueberries
- 1½ cups coconut milk
- ¼ cup maple syrup
- ¼ teaspoon cinnamon
- ⅛ teaspoon salt

1. In a small bowl, roughly mash the blueberries.
2. Divide the blueberry mixture among 6 ice pop molds.
3. In a medium bowl, mix together the coconut milk, maple syrup, cinnamon, and salt.
4. Pour the coconut milk mixture into the ice pop molds over the blueberries.
5. Freeze for at least 2 hours, or until solid.

PER SERVING:

Calories: 186| Total Fat: 14g| Total Carbohydrates: 16g| Sugar: 12g| Fiber: 2g| Protein: 2g| Sodium: 37mg

Almond Butter and Chocolate Cookies

Prep time: 5 minutes | **Cook time:** 15 minutes | **Serves 8**

- 1 stick butter
- 1/2 cup almond butter
- 1/2 cup Monk fruit powder
- 3 cups pork rinds, crushed
- 1 teaspoon vanilla extract
- 1/4 teaspoon ground cinnamon
- 1/2 cup sugar-free chocolate, cut into chunks
- 1/2 cup double cream

1. In a pan, melt the butter, almond butter, and Monk fruit powder over medium heat.
2. Now, add the crushed pork rinds and vanilla. Place the batter on a cookie sheet and let it cool in your refrigerator.
3. Meanwhile, in a small saucepan over medium heat, melt the chocolate and double cream. Add the chocolate layer over the batter.
4. Allow it to chill completely before slicing and serving. Bon appétit!

PER SERVING

Calories: 322 | Fat: 28.9g | Carbs: 3.4g | Fiber: 0.6g | Protein: 13.9g

Basic Orange Cheesecake

Prep time: 5 minutes | Cook time:15 minutes |Serves 12

- 1 tablespoon Swerve
- 1 cup almond flour
- 1 stick butter, room temperature 1/2 cup unsweetened coconut, shredded
- Filling:
- 1 teaspoon powdered gelatin
- 2 tablespoons Swerve
- 17 ounces mascarpone cream
- 2 tablespoon orange juice

1. Thoroughly combine all the ingredients for the crust; press the crust mixture into a lightly greased baking dish.
2. Let it stand in your refrigerator.
3. Then, mix 1 cup of boiling water and gelatin until all dissolved. Pour in 1 cup of cold water.
4. Add Swerve, mascarpone cheese, and orange juice; blend until smooth and uniform. Pour the filling onto the prepared crust. Enjoy!

PER SERVING

Calories: 150 | Fat: 15.4g | Carbs: 2.1g | Fiber: 0.1g |Protein: 1.2g

Peanut Butter and Chocolate Treat

Prep time: 5 minutes | Cook time:10 minutes | Serves 10

- 1 stick butter, room temperature
- 1/3 cup peanut butter
- 1/3 cup unsweetened cocoa powder
- 1/3 cup Swerve
- 1/2 teaspoon ground cinnamon
- A pinch of grated nutmeg
- 1/4 cup unsweetened coconut flakes
- 1/4 cup pork rinds, crushed

1. Melt the butter and peanut butter until smooth and uniform.
2. Add the remaining ingredients and mix until everything is well combined.
3. Line a baking sheet with a silicone baking mat. Pour the mixture into the baking sheet. Place in your freezer for 1 hour until ready to serve. Enjoy!

PER SERVING

Calories: 122 | Fat: 11.7g | Carbs: 4.9g | Fiber: 1.4g | Protein: 1.5g

Peanut and Butter Cubes

Prep time: 5 minutes | Cook time:50 minutes |Serves 10

- 1 stick butter
- 1/3 cup coconut oil
- 1 vanilla paste
- 1/4 teaspoon cinnamon powder
- 2 tablespoons Monk fruit powder
- A pinch of coarse salt
- 1/2 cup peanuts, toasted and coarsely chopped

1. Microwave the butter, coconut oil, and vanilla until melted. Add cinnamon powder, Monk fruit powder, and salt.
2. Put the chopped peanuts into a silicon mold or an ice cube tray. Pour the warm butter mixture over the peanuts.
3. Place in your freezer for 40 to 50 minutes. Bon appétit!

PER SERVING

Calories: 218 | Fat: 21.2g | Carbs: 5.1g | Fiber: 0.7g | Protein: 3.8g

Carrot Nori Rolls

Prep time: 5 minutes | Cook time: 10 minutes | Serves 4

- 2 tbsp almond butter
- 2 tbsp tamari
- 4 standard nori sheets
- 1 green bell pepper, sliced
- 1 tbsp pickled ginger
- ½ cup grated carrots

1. Preheat your oven to 350°F.
2. Whisk the almond butter and tamari until smooth and thick.
3. Place a nori sheet on a flat surface with the rough side facing up.
4. Spoon a bit of the tamari mixture at the other side of the nori sheet, and spread on all sides.
5. Put bell pepper slices, carrots, and ginger in a layer at the other end of the sheet.
6. Fold up in the tahini direction to seal.
7. Repeat the process with the remaining sheets.
8. Arrange on a baking tray and bake for about 10 minutes until browned and crispy.
9. Allow cooling for a few minutes before slicing into 4 pieces.

PER SERVING

Cal 70| Fat 6g| Carbs 3g| Protein 1g

Coconut Cranberry Bars

Prep time: 5 minutes | Cook time: 1 hour 10 minutes |Serves 12

- 1/3 cup cranberries
- 1 ½ cups coconut flakes, unsweetened
- 1/2 cup butter, melted
- 1/2 teaspoon liquid Stevia

1. Mix all ingredients in your food processor until well combined. Press the batter into a baking sheet.
2. Refrigerate for 1 hour. Cut into bars and serve well chilled.

PER SERVING

Calories: 107 | Fat: 11.1g | Carbs: 2.5g | Fiber: 0.9g | Protein: 0.4g

Mediterranean Tahini Beans

Prep time: 5 minutes | Cook time: 5 minutes | Serves 4

- 1 tbsp extra-virgin olive oil
- 1 cup string beans, trimmed
- Sea salt to taste
- 2 tbsp pure tahini
- 2 tbsp chopped mint leaves
- ¼ tsp red chili flakes

1. Pour the string beans into a microwave dish, sprinkle with 1 tbsp of water, and steam in the microwave until softened, 1 minute.
2. Heat the olive oil in a large skillet and toss in the string beans until well coated in the butter.
3. Season with salt and mix in the tahini and mint leaves.
4. Cook for 1-2 minutes.
5. Serve immediately.

PER SERVING

Cal 80| Fat 5g| Carbs 10g| Protein 1g

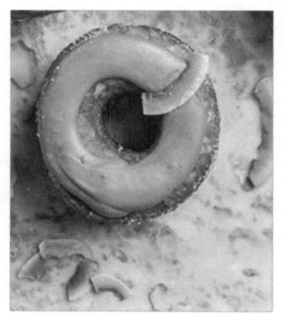

Pepita Cheese Tomato Chips

Prep time: 5 minutes | Cook time: 10 minutes | Serves 6

- 5 tomatoes, sliced
- ¼ cup extra-virgin olive oil
- ½ cup pepitas seeds
- 1 tbsp nutritional yeast
- Sea salt and pepper to taste
- 1 tsp garlic puree

1. Preheat your oven to 400°F.
2. Over the sliced tomatoes, drizzle olive oil.
3. In a food processor, add pepitas seeds, nutritional yeast, garlic, salt, and pepper and pulse until the desired consistency is attained.
4. Toss in tomato slices to coat.
5. Set the tomato slices on a baking pan and bake for 10 minutes.
6. Serve and enjoy!

PER SERVING

Cal 150| Fat 14g| Carbs 6g| Protein 4g

Easiest Brownies Ever

Prep time: 5 minutes | Cook time: 1 hour |Serves 10

- 2 tablespoons almond flour
- 3 tablespoons coconut flour
- 1/2 teaspoon baking powder
- 1/2 cup cocoa powder, unsweetened
- 4 eggs
- 1/2 cup Swerve
- 1 teaspoon almond extract
- 1 vanilla extract
- 1/2 cup coconut oil
- 3 ounces baking chocolate, unsweetened

1. Thoroughly combine the almond flour, coconut flour, cocoa powder, and baking powder.
2. Mix in the eggs, Swerve, almond and vanilla extract; beat with an electric mixer on high until everything is well combined.
3. In a separate bowl, melt the coconut oil and chocolate in your microwave. Now, add the egg mixture and mix again.
4. Gradually add the dry ingredients and whisk until everything is well incorporated. Pour the batter into a lightly greased baking pan.
5. Bake in the preheated oven at 320 degrees F approximately 50 minutes or until a toothpick inserted into the middle of your brownie comes out clean and dry. Bon appétit!

PER SERVING

Calories: 205 | Fat: 19.5g | Carbs: 5.4g | Fiber: 3.2g | Protein: 4.7g

No Bake Party Cake

Prep time: 10 minutes | Cook time:30 minutes |Serves 6

- 1/4 cup almond flour
- 1/4 cup coconut flour
- 2 tablespoons cocoa powder
- 1½ tablespoons Swerve
- 1 tablespoon almond butter
- 2 tablespoons coconut oilA pinch of salt
- A pinch of cinnamon powder
- 7 ounces mascarpone cheese
- 2 tablespoons coconut oil
- 2 tablespoons cocoa powder
- 1/4 cup tablespoons Swerve
- 1/3 cup double cream
- 2 tablespoons Irish whiskey
- 1 teaspoon vanilla extract
- 1/2 cup double cream
- 1 teaspoon grass-fed gelatin

1. In a small bowl, thoroughly combine the almond flour, coconut flour, cocoa, and Swerve.
2. Add almond butter, coconut oil, salt, and cinnamon powder; press the crust into a baking pan.
3. To make the filling, melt mascarpone cheese and coconut oil in a microwave for 40 seconds.
4. Add cocoa, Swerve, 1/3 cup of cream, Irish whiskey, and vanilla; beat with an electric mixer until creamy and uniform.
5. Then, whip 1/2 cup of double cream until it has doubled in volume.
6. In a small mixing bowl, combine gelatin with 1 tablespoon of cold water; whisk until dissolved. Now, add 1 tablespoon of hot water and stir until well combined.
7. Slowly and gradually, add dissolved gelatin to the whipped cream; mix until stiff. Now, fold the prepared whipped cream into the cream cheese mixture.
8. Spread the filling over the crust and serve well chilled. Enjoy!

PER SERVING

Calories: 274 | Fat: 27.5g | Carbs: 5.7g | Fiber: 1.6g | Protein: 3.8g

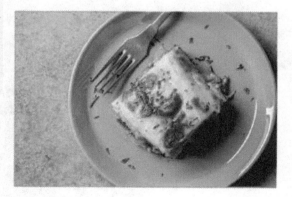

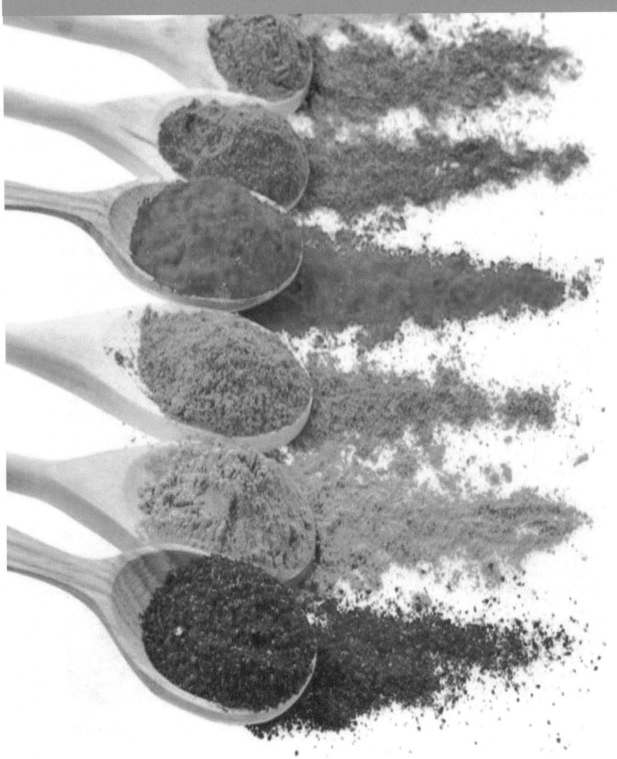

Creamy Coconut Herb Dressing

Prep time: 5 minutes | Cook time: 40-45 minutes | Makes 1 cup

- 8 ounces plain coconut yogurt
- 2 tablespoons freshly squeezed lemon juice
- 2 tablespoons chopped fresh parsley
- 1 tablespoon snipped fresh chives
- ½ teaspoon salt
- Pinch freshly ground black pepper

1. In a medium bowl, whisk together the yogurt, lemon juice, parsley, chives, salt, and pepper.
2. Refrigerate in an airtight container.

PER SERVING

Calories: 14 | Total Fat: 1g | Total Carbohydrates: 2g | Sugar: 0g | Fiber: 1g | Protein: 0g | Sodium: 172mg

Avocado Dressing

Prep time: 10 minutes | Cook time: 40-45 minutes | Makes 2 cups

- 1 ripe avocado
- 1 cup plain coconut yogurt
- ¼ cup freshly squeezed lemon juice
- 1 scallion, chopped
- 1 tablespoon chopped fresh cilantro

1. In a food processor, blend the avocado, yogurt, lemon juice, scallion, and cilantro until smooth.
2. Refrigerate in an airtight container.

PER SERVING

Calories: 33 | Total Fat: 3g | Total Carbohydrates: 2g | Sugar: 0g | Fiber: 1g | Protein: 0g | Sodium: 14mg

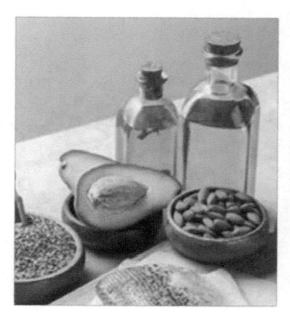

Cherry-Peach Chutney with Mint

Prep time: 15 minutes | Cook time: 15 minutes | Makes 2 cups

- 1 (10-ounce) bag frozen no-added-sugar peach chunks, thawed, drained, coarsely chopped, juice reserved
- ½ medium red onion, diced
- ¼ cup dried cherries, coarsely chopped
- 2 tablespoons freshly squeezed lemon juice
- 1 tablespoon raw honey or maple syrup
- 1 teaspoon apple cider vinegar
- ¼ teaspoon salt
- 1 tablespoon chopped fresh mint leaves

1. Place the peach chunks in a medium bowl.
2. Stir in the onion, cherries, lemon juice, honey, cider vinegar, and salt.
3. Let the mixture stand for 30 minutes before serving.
4. When ready to serve, stir in the mint.
5. Refrigerate in an airtight container for no more than three days.

PER SERVING

Calories: 42 | Total Fat: 0g | Total Carbohydrates: 10g | Sugar: 7g | Fiber: 2g | Protein: 1g | Sodium: 76mg

Fiesta Guacamole

Prep time: 15 minutes | Cook time: 15 minutes | Makes 3 cups

- 3 medium Hass avocados, halved, pitted, and peeled
- 3 small radishes, sliced
- 3 large strawberries, diced
- 3 cloves garlic, minced
- 1 green onion, sliced
- ½ bunch fresh cilantro (about 1½ ounces), minced
- Juice of 2 lemons
- 2 teaspoons fine Himalayan salt
- 1 tablespoon extra-virgin olive oil

1. Place all the ingredients in a large bowl. Use a whisk or pestle to mix and mash them together until you have a chunky guacamole.
2. If it's not all going to be consumed right away, transfer it to an airtight container, drizzle olive oil on it, set a sheet of plastic wrap on the top so that it sticks directly to the guacamole—this will help keep the avocado from turning brown—and then put the lid on. Store in the fridge until ready to enjoy, but no more than 4 days.

PER SERVING

Calories: 215 | Fat: 18 g | Total Carbohydrate: 15g | Dietary Fiber: 9g | Protein: 4g

Berry Vinaigrette

Prep time: 15 minutes | Cook time: 15 minutes | Makes 1 ½ cups

- 1 cup berries, fresh or frozen, no added sugar (thawed if frozen)
- ½ cup balsamic vinegar
- ⅓ cup extra-virgin olive oil
- 2 tablespoons freshly squeezed lemon or lime juice
- 1 tablespoon raw honey or maple syrup
- 1 tablespoon lemon or lime zest
- 1 tablespoon Dijon mustard
- 1 teaspoon salt
- ½ teaspoon freshly ground black pepper

1. In a blender, purée the berries, balsamic vinegar, olive oil, lemon juice, honey, lemon zest, Dijon mustard, salt, and pepper until smooth.
2. Refrigerate in an airtight container for up to five days.

PER SERVING

Calories: 73 | Total Fat: 7g | Total Carbohydrates: 3g | Sugar: 2g | Fiber: 0g | Protein: 0g | Sodium: 210mg

Honey-Mustard Sesame Sauce

Prep time: 10 minutes | Cook time: 15 minutes |Makes 1 cup

- ½ cup Dijon mustard
- ½ cup raw honey or maple syrup
- 1 garlic clove, minced
- 1 teaspoon toasted sesame oil

1. In a small bowl, whisk together the Dijon, honey, garlic, and sesame oil.
2. Refrigerate in an airtight container.

PER SERVING

Calories: 67 | Total Fat: 1g | Total Carbohydrates: 14g | Sugar: 12g | Fiber: 1g | Protein: 1g | Sodium: 179mg

Almost Caesar Salad Dressing

Prep time: 10 minutes | Cook time: 15 minutes | Makes 1 cup

- ¾ cup extra-virgin olive oil
- 3 tablespoons apple cider vinegar
- 2 anchovy fillets
- ½ teaspoon salt
- Freshly ground black pepper

1. In a blender or food processor, purée the olive oil, cider vinegar, anchovies, garlic, salt, and pepper until smooth.
2. Refrigerate in an airtight container and use within one week.

PER SERVING

Calories: 166 | Total Fat: 19g | Total Carbohydrates: 0g | Sugar: 0g | Fiber: 0g | Protein: 0g | Sodium: 184mg

Cauliflower Alfredo

Prep time: 10 minutes | Cook time: 15 minutes | Makes 2 cups

- 3 cups cauliflower florets
- 5 cloves garlic, peeled
- 1 cup full-fat coconut milk
- 3 tablespoons salted butter, ghee, or lard
- 1 tablespoon fish sauce
- 1 tablespoon red wine vinegar
- 1 teaspoon fine Himalayan salt
- 1 teaspoon ground black pepper

1. Fill a saucepan with about an inch of water and add the cauliflower and garlic. Heat the pan over medium-high heat and bring to a boil with the lid on. Cook for about 8 minutes, until the cauliflower is fork-tender. Remove from the heat and drain.
2. Place the cauliflower, garlic, and remaining ingredients in a blender. Puree until smooth.
3. Store in an airtight container in the fridge for up to 10 days. To reheat, bring to a simmer in a saucepan over medium heat.

PER SERVING

Calories: 250 | Fat: 24 g | Total Carbohydrate: 9 g | Dietary Fiber: 3.4g | Protein: 3.5g

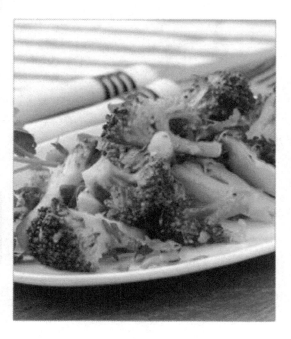

Pickled Red Onions

Prep time: 5 minutes, plus 30 minutes to steep | Cook time: 15 minutes | Makes 4 cups

- 2 cups filtered water
- 1 cup apple cider vinegar
- 1 teaspoon fine Himalayan salt
- 1 teaspoon granulated erythritol or other low-carb sweetener (optional; see Note)
- 2 bay leaves
- 2 red onions, thinly sliced and cut into half-moons
- Special equipment:
- 3 cup or larger glass or ceramic container with a tight-fitting lid

1. Combine the water, vinegar, salt, erythritol (if using), and bay leaves in a small saucepan over medium heat. Bring to a light simmer and cook for about 8 minutes. Stir to make sure the salt and sweetener have dissolved.
2. Put all the onion slices in a jar with the bay leaves and then pour the hot brine over the onions until they are fully submerged. Let the onions steep for 30 minutes at room temperature before using. Seal the jar and store in the fridge for up to 1 month.

PER SERVING

Calories: 5 | Fat: 0g | Total Carbohydrate: 2g | Dietary Fiber: 0.2g | Protein: 0g

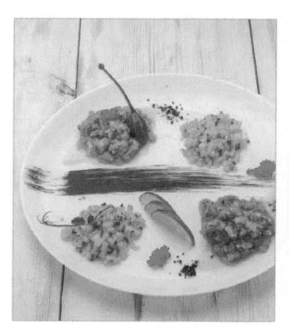

Everything Bacon

Prep time: 5 minutes | Cook time: 15 minutes | Serves 5

- 10 slices bacon
- 1 teaspoon dried dill weed
- 1 teaspoon onion powder
- 1 teaspoon poppy seeds
- 1 teaspoon toasted sesame seeds
- ¼ teaspoon fine Himalayan salt

1. Lay the slices of bacon flat on a sheet pan. Sprinkle the seasonings evenly over the bacon. The higher up you sprinkle from, the more evenly the bacon will be seasoned.
2. Place the sheet pan in the oven and set the temperature to 375°F. (Note: Don't preheat the oven! You want to start with a cold oven.) Bake until the oven comes to temperature, then for 10 to 15 minutes more. (I like to make this bacon extra crispy; if you prefer softer bacon, take it out of the oven sooner.) Keep an eye on it for the last few minutes. When it's ready, it will be dark brown and firm, and your home will smell of bacon.
3. Store flat in an airtight container in the fridge for up to 8 days. Bring to room temperature before adding to salads or snacking on, and heat in a warm skillet before adding to hot dishes.

PER SERVING

Calories: 214 | Fat: 16.5g | Total Carbohydrate: 1.3g | Dietary Fiber: 0.2g | Protein: 14.4g

Ranch Dressing

Prep time: 5 minutes | Cook time: 15 minutes | Makes 1½ cups

- ½ cup filtered water
- ½ cup shelled hemp seeds (aka hemp hearts)
- 2 tablespoons red wine vinegar
- 1 tablespoon coconut aminos (optional)
- 1 tablespoon Dijon mustard
- 2 teaspoons dried dill weed
- 1 teaspoon dried parsley
- 1 teaspoon fine Himalayan salt
- 1 teaspoon garlic powder
- 1 teaspoon onion powder
- 1 teaspoon ground black pepper

1. Place all of the ingredients in a blender and blend until smooth.
2. Store in an airtight glass or ceramic container in the fridge for up to 10 days. Set out at room temperature to soften for a few minutes before using, and shake or stir to mix well.

PER SERVING

Calories: 225 | Fat: 18g | Total Carbohydrate: 4g | Dietary Fiber: 2.2g | Protein: 10.7g

Appendix 1 Measurement Conversion Chart

Volume Equivalents (Dry)	
US STANDARD	METRIC (APPROXIMATE)
1/8 teaspoon	0.5 mL
1/4 teaspoon	1 mL
1/2 teaspoon	2 mL
3/4 teaspoon	4 mL
1 teaspoon	5 mL
1 tablespoon	15 mL
1/4 cup	59 mL
1/2 cup	118 mL
3/4 cup	177 mL
1 cup	235 mL
2 cups	475 mL
3 cups	700 mL
4 cups	1 L

Volume Equivalents (Liquid)		
US STANDARD	US STANDARD (OUNCES)	METRIC (APPROXIMATE)
2 tablespoons	1 fl.oz.	30 mL
1/4 cup	2 fl.oz.	60 mL
1/2 cup	4 fl.oz.	120 mL
1 cup	8 fl.oz.	240 mL
1 1/2 cup	12 fl.oz.	355 mL
2 cups or 1 pint	16 fl.oz.	475 mL
4 cups or 1 quart	32 fl.oz.	1 L
1 gallon	128 fl.oz.	4 L

Weight Equivalents	
US STANDARD	METRIC (APPROXIMATE)
1 ounce	28 g
2 ounces	57 g
5 ounces	142 g
10 ounces	284 g
15 ounces	425 g
16 ounces (1 pound)	455 g
1.5 pounds	680 g
2 pounds	907 g

Temperatures Equivalents	
FAHRENHEIT(F)	CELSIUS(C) APPROXIMATE)
225 °F	107 °C
250 °F	120 ° °C
275 °F	135 °C
300 °F	150 °C
325 °F	160 °C
350 °F	180 °C
375 °F	190 °C
400 °F	205 °C
425 °F	220 °C
450 °F	235 °C
475 °F	245 °C
500 °F	260 °C

Appendix 2 The Dirty Dozen and Clean Fifteen

The Environmental Working Group (EWG) is a nonprofit, nonpartisan organization dedicated to protecting human health and the environment Its mission is to empower people to live healthier lives in a healthier environment. This organization publishes an annual list of the twelve kinds of produce, in sequence, that have the highest amount of pesticide residue-the Dirty Dozen-as well as a list of the fifteen kinds ofproduce that have the least amount of pesticide residue-the Clean Fifteen.

THE DIRTY DOZEN	
The 2016 Dirty Dozen includes the following produce. These are considered among the year's most important produce to buy organic:	
Strawberries	Spinach
Apples	Tomatoes
Nectarines	Bell peppers
Peaches	Cherry tomatoes
Celery	Cucumbers
Grapes	Kale/collard greens
Cherries	Hot peppers
The Dirty Dozen list contains two additional itemskale/collard greens and hot peppers-because they tend to contain trace levels of highly hazardous pesticides.	

THE CLEAN FIFTEEN	
The least critical to buy organically are the Clean Fifteen list. The following are on the 2016 list:	
Avocados	Papayas
Corn	Kiw
Pineapples	Eggplant
Cabbage	Honeydew
Sweet peas	Grapefruit
Onions	Cantaloupe
Asparagus	Cauliflower
Mangos	
Some of the sweet corn sold in the United States are made from genetically engineered (GE) seedstock. Buy organic varieties of these crops to avoid GE produce.	

Appendix 3 Index

MARY D. NELSON

Made in the USA
Las Vegas, NV
11 October 2023